Energy Medicine

*This book is dedicated
to
Nora
Alvah
and the wonderful spirit
of
Will*

For Churchill Livingstone:

Editorial Director:	Mary Law
Project Development Manager:	Valerie Dearing
Project Manager:	Jane Shanks
Design Direction:	George Ajayi

Energy Medicine
The Scientific Basis

James L. Oschman PhD
Nature's Own Research Association
Dover
New Hampshire
USA

Foreword by
Candace Pert PhD
Research Professor
Department of Physiology and Biophysics
Georgetown University School of Medicine
Washington, DC
USA

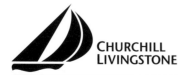

CHURCHILL
LIVINGSTONE

EDINBURGH LONDON NEW YORK OXFORD PHILADELPHIA ST LOUIS SYDNEY TORONTO 2000

CHURCHILL LIVINGSTONE
An imprint of Elsevier Limited

First published 2000
  Reprinted 2000, 2001, 2002 (twice), 2003, 2004 (twice)

ISBN 0 443 06261 7

British Library Cataloguing in Publication Data
A catalogue record for this book is available from the British Library.

Library of Congress Cataloging in Publication Data
A catalog record for this book is available from the Library of Congress.

Note
Medical knowledge is constantly changing. As new information
becomes available, changes in treatment, procedures, equipment and
the use of drugs become necessary. The author and the publishers
have, as far as it is possible, taken care to ensure that the information
given in this text is accurate and up to date. However, readers are
strongly advised to confirm that the information, especially with
regard to drug usage, complies with the latest legislation and standards
of practice.

 your source for books,
journals and multimedia
in the health sciences
www.elsevierhealth.com

The
publisher's
policy is to use
paper manufactured
from sustainable forests

Printed in China
C/08

Contents

Foreword

For a number of years before I actually had the profound pleasure of meeting Dr Oschman, I kept hearing about him from energy therapists of many types. Here was a real scientist, a cellular biologist and physiologist with impeccable credentials, who dared to associate with Rolfers, acupuncturists and other bodyworkers in a bold search to establish the nature of the real science underlying energy medicine. Dr Oschman's quest was to explain and document what he had learned with clarity and scholarship in such a convincing way that old paradigm naysayers would be forced to listen and join the dialog. Now he has succeeded by providing us with a breakthrough text which maps out an elegant theory of the human body and how it is impacted upon by energy medicine. This is a theory fully compatible with classical physiological and electromagnetic principles, as well as electronics and modern physics, a theory which doesn't need to invoke 'subtle energies' or other mysterious forces which currently lack a scientific rationale.

For years I had lectured and written on the power of healing techniques considered at best unorthodox and at worst quackish, which I had experienced in my own body as powerful and having merit despite the strong resistance and irrational dismissal by most of conventional medicine and my own inability to explain them in the conventional biological paradigm. Feeling 'energy moving' is a common denominator in many of these techniques and I constantly experienced this from my first encounter with acupuncture over twenty-five years ago to my recent interaction with Dr Oschman at the AMTA (American Massage Therapy Association) meeting to design scientific experiments to demonstrate the efficacy and mechanism of action of massage therapy. There in South Carolina, when Dr Oschman proceeded to 'pull' some energy away from my 'stagnant' liver, I felt the appropriate movement before he had even described it. Thus in scientific parlance I was blind to the anticipated outcome, as when years earlier my young son, unaware of the reflexology chart, had accurately reeled off six or seven places in his body to where he had felt 'something move' from the six or seven points of his feet I had manipulated in accordance with that chart. These types of mini-experiment on myself and family over the years had convinced me that there is something so compelling that energy medicine should be taken seriously and studied, not squelched and ignored simply because the reigning paradigm – until now – had no theories to explain it.

How exciting then that Dr Oschman's research has provided a brilliant, concise simple explanation for the sense shared in many diverse energy therapies that claim that energy must move in the body. Today most bodyworkers and body psychotherapists take as a fact the twin neo-Freudian and neo-Reichian concepts that trauma is absorbed and stored in the body and can be unblocked by some corrective energy flow. I have understood for some time that therapeutic massage can be so much more than increasing the blood circulation in sore muscles; our concept of the psychosomatic network (Pert 1999) envisions memories stored in the body (the subconscious mind) in the form of alterations at receptor molecules which transduce chemical changes into ionic fluxes and thus the propagation of electromagnetic waves throughout the network which joins the nervous system, immune cells, gut, glands, skin, etc.

Dr Oschman carefully traces the history of ideas from several fields which support his vision of the body as a liquid crystal under tension capable of vibrating at a number of frequencies, some in the range of visible light. Based upon these revolutionary, but well-supported ideas, I am most excited about the new possibilities of bringing about a rigorous understanding of the nature of emotions on an energetic level. In emphasizing emotions as the mind–body bridge, I have been struck by the ability to span the physical realm of internal communication via ligands and receptors and the spiritual realm of external communication among people, animals and the rest of nature. It will be most interesting to begin to gain more experimental proof of the external energetic patterns emitted from the hands of healers, the approach Dr Oschman was recommending in South Carolina. We can then start to attempt to measure and understand the energetic forces that act together on seemingly separate creatures which in reality must be continually subjected to unifying emotional(?) forces which drive them to interact more like molecules in solution.

It is not difficult now to imagine different emotional states, each with a pre-dominant peptide ligand-induced 'tone' as an energetic pattern which propagates throughout the bodymind, a 'vibratory flow' which can restore communication among 'blocked', diseased or unintegrated body parts. I too have moved beyond the 'lock and key' model of receptor/ligand binding to the notion of vibrating receptors and ligands which attract at a distance as they resonate at the same frequency. Dr Oschman's new paradigm vision of the human body allows me at last to be able to begin to understand how different emotional states, by triggering the release of various peptide ligands, trigger sudden, even quantum, shifts in consciousness accompanied by concomitant shifts in behavior, memory and body posture. Perhaps we can now begin to imagine how physical 'adjustments' of spinal joints that house peptidergic nerve bundles, therapies that emphasize emotional expression and feeling within the body, and hands on healings where practitioners claim to be able to feel energetic differences and emit appropriate corrective energies share common energetic mechanisms.

The publication of *Energy Medicine – The Scientific Basis* by Jim Oschman is a milestone in the history of medicine which will open hearts and minds to new hypotheses and experimental approaches toward understanding important modes of healing previously thought to be too mysterious to be approached scientifically. Also, we may begin to have a new paradigm vision of the human body as a dynamic shape-shifting bundle of multiple personalities, not merely layered, but capable of sudden and dramatic transformations able to be stabilized in new healing states of mind and body. Bravo!

Candace B. Pert

Reference

Pert C 1999 Molecules of emotion: the science behind mind–body medicine. Simon & Schuster, New York

Preface

This book is about a subject that scientists have always found extremely controversial and confusing. For centuries, concepts of 'life force' and 'healing energy' have been virtually off-limits for consideration by serious and respectable scientists. Therapeutic approaches employing healing energy have been regarded with a great deal of skepticism. The legacy of this history is that there are many who will not even open a book such as this.

Why, then, would a serious and thoughtful scientist dare to take on this subject? Those willing to read on will find that there are extraordinarily good reasons. Stated simply, times have changed dramatically. Both scientists and energy therapists around the world have made discoveries that have forever altered our picture of human energetics. Individually, most of these discoveries have not been perceived as major breakthroughs or milestones. But it now appears that the seemingly disparate experimental results and experiences and concepts are converging. A promising new branch of academic inquiry and clinical research is opening up. Approaches that have appeared in competition or conflict are actually supporting each other.

The book is the outcome of an invitation by Dr Leon Chaitow and his editorial team at the *Journal of Bodywork and Movement Therapies*, published by Churchill Livingstone, an imprint of Harcourt Publishers. I was asked to clarify and come to terms with the word 'energy' as it is utilized both in science and in the various branches of bodywork and movement therapies, and in health care generally (Magnetic Resonance Imaging (MRI) scans for example). Was 'energy' a concept that could be explained in terms acceptable to a scientific and intellectually critical mind?

I had already researched this topic for about 15 years: the invitation from Dr Chaitow gave me an opportunity to gather together many more pieces of a fascinating puzzle.

In the process of writing the journal articles, I noticed similarities between the discoveries of modern medical researchers and the daily observations of 'hands-on' energy therapists. In essence, these traditionally very different approaches to the body are beginning to validate one another.

To be specific, and to anticipate Chapter 6, oscillating magnetic fields are being researched at various medical centers for the treatment of bone, nerve, skin, capillary, and ligament damage. Virtually identical energy fields can also be detected around the hands of suitably trained therapists. There is an inescapable conclusion:

Medical research is demonstrating that devices producing pulsing magnetic fields of particular frequencies can stimulate the healing of a variety of tissues. Therapists from various schools of energy medicine can project, from their hands, fields with similar frequencies and intensities. Research documenting that these different approaches are efficacious is mutually validating. Medical research and hands-on therapies are confirming each other. The common denominator is the pulsating magnetic field, which is called a biomagnetic field when it emanates from the hands of a therapist.

In addition, Dr Chaitow asked me to describe how the evolving concepts might impact specific clinical practices. The inclusion of clinical aspects added a valuable focus to the articles. An appreciation of current energy medicine research enables students and practitioners of all therapeutic disciplines to find a common ground for discussion. Complementary therapies complement each other. Phenomena that previously seemed disconnected could supplement one another, leading to a better understanding of the living body than would be achieved by any single approach. I thank Dr Chaitow for having the foresight to set this rewarding process in motion.

This book gives me the opportunity to include details that could not be fitted into the journal articles because of space constraints. It also enables me to bring the story up to date with discoveries that have been made since the articles were written. In this book, I have expanded on important topics that were only mentioned in the journal articles, such as emerging information on the physics underlying energy, and the roles of energy in consciousness. Finally, it is possible to include a wealth of technical information and quotations that was not appropriate for the journal. This material will be of particular interest to the professional scientist wishing to critique the ideas presented here. Some of this information is technical, and the non-technical reader can skip it if they wish.

Only passing reference is made to the ways that various energy techniques are practiced and to the extensive and growing research that supports their claims of clinical efficacy. The reader interested in these topics can consult the appropriate schools that teach clinical techniques, and the relevant clinical literature. My inquiry is an attempt to use the latest scientific research to answer the question 'If it works then how does it work?' An understanding of mechanisms is crucial, because successful clinical trials have much more impact if there is a logical explanation of how a method works. Moreover, therapists benefit enormously from knowledge of mechanisms, as it helps them explain and even enhance their work.

I have received treatments from practitioners of many of the techniques described, and I am convinced that these experiences have helped me become more aware of myself and of my personal energy system. However, I am not an advocate of any one method over another. I have lectured at various schools of bodywork and movement therapy around the world, but am not on the faculty of any of them. The aim here is not to promote any particular method, but to help understand the mechanisms involved and connect the phenomena with medical science. We have much to learn from each other if we can learn to use a common language.

I thank all of the clinicians who have challenged me to explain their insights and observations. Peter Melchior started me on this journey, by telling me details of important scientific research – such as that of Dr Harold Saxton Burr – that I had never encountered during my academic education. Dr Chaitow and the staff of Churchill Livingstone did an excellent job of producing the series for the *Journal of Bodywork and Movement Therapies*, and Graeme Chambers efficiently and professionally rendered the artwork. I particularly thank the production editors, Lynn Percy and Ewan Halley, and the copy-editor, Sally Livitt, for their careful work in preparing the manuscripts for publication in the journal, and Stephanie Pickering for her thorough editing of the book manuscript. I am indebted to the many scientists and therapists who have alerted me to important discoveries so that I can include them in this book. And I am especially appreciative of the role of my dear wife, Nora, who knows more about energy than I ever will. She discussed every aspect of this work with me, and gave me the freedom and encouragement to wander deeply into the minutest nooks and crannies of living structure and energy.

Dover, New Hampshire, 2000   James L. Oschman

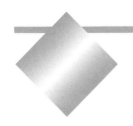

Introduction

This book tells two stories. One is the story of the emergence of a new and tremendously exciting branch of academic medicine. Behind this emerging science is the equally fascinating tale of why the whole subject has been so confusing and controversial in the past. This second narrative accounts for the paradox of the enduring and widespread academic skepticism and myopia about therapeutic approaches that are based on concepts of energy, at the same time that these methods appear to be benefiting many people.

Many therapists who work daily and successfully with human energy systems have felt alienated from the sciences that provide the logical and rational foundation for conventional medicine. Some of their most remarkable and important experiences, and those of their clients, seem to defy analysis from current scientific perspectives. A close look at energy medicine resolves this unnecessary confusion and controversy.

Over the last few decades, scientists have developed more than adequate measurable and logical connections between biological energy fields and generally accepted scientific knowledge. Methods have been developed to measure subtle but important energy fields within and around the human body. A few decades ago these fields were considered nonexistent by academic medicine. Not only are we documenting the presence of such fields, but researchers are understanding how fields are generated and how they are altered by disease and disorder. We are also beginning to understand the biophysical mechanisms that enable the discerning therapist to sense and manipulate energy fields for the benefit of the patient.

In essence, a major gap in biology is being filled. The new discoveries are not being developed within any particular discipline or by a particular method. Instead, fundamental observations are being made in a wide variety of areas. After all, like it or not, any approach to the body utilizes energy in one form or another. An open-minded consideration of energetics has the potential to improve the treatment of serious disorders and diseases that do not respond to clinical methods based on concepts that leave energy out of the picture.

We now know that the living organism is designed both to adapt to and utilize many different kinds of forces, and that healing processes involve the operation of many kinds of communications. There is no single 'life force' or 'healing energy.' Instead, there are many systems in the body that conduct various kinds of energy and information from place to place. Different energetic therapies focus on different aspects of this multiplicity, and each of these therapies presents a valuable set of clues and testable hypotheses about how human energy systems work. The physiological and anatomical systems in the body and the energy systems interdigitate. Effective therapeutic work on one system inevitably affects the composite.

Energetics is therefore a rich multi-disciplinary topic. Following the flows of energy through the body is a lesson in every domain of biology, ranging from geophysical to inter-organismal interactions (the ecological level) to physiology and behavior, organs, tissues, cells, molecules, atoms, and subatomic particles. This is a rich and fascinating perspective for exploration. Not only does energy teach us about the minutest parts of the living body, but also energetic interactions account for the important properties that arise from the relations between the parts. One of these properties we call wholeness, the integration that enables the parts to work together as a successful unit.

This book is a 'snapshot' of a scene that is rapidly coming into focus. Fundamental discoveries are reported almost daily. In the process, many observations and experiences that have defied explanation in the past are being demystified. So much information is emerging that it is challenging for a single individual to keep track of all of it. As a result some important discoveries are undoubtedly missing from these pages, simply because of this fact.

Discoveries on energetics are gradually percolating into the consciousness of conventional medical practitioners and researchers. As our knowledge of energy biology is refined, it becomes easier to explore and manipulate living energy systems, and to explain what is happening to the curious and interested – and often delighted – patient. A major impetus is the recognition among both health care professionals and the general public that complementary medicine and energy therapies are here to stay, and that these methods can often help the patient who has not found relief from more orthodox approaches.

While this book was in preparation, a number of therapists published fascinating descriptions of the ways their work is being incorporated into hospitals and clinics. Among these is the work of Julie Motz (1998) and her physician colleague, Mehmet Oz (1998). Others have written compelling books about their personal experiences with energy healing (eg Collinge 1998, Egidio 1997, Brennan 1987). I mention these sources because I believe the experiences they describe, extraordinary as they may sometimes seem, lay a foundation for future medical inquiries into energy biology: 'The scientist knows that in the history of ideas, magic always precedes science, that the intuition of phenomena anticipates their objective knowledge' (Gauguelin 1974).

Energetic medicine is pointing in an obvious direction. Most of us prefer a personal philosophy and a medicine that enables us to get over our physical or emotional sicknesses or injuries immediately, if not sooner. The phenomenon of 'spontaneous remission' is a dramatic indication of our innate potential to recover from the most devastating conditions. Clinical experience has shown that rapid and spontaneous remissions can and do happen, even for the most potent cancers or for the most catastrophic of injuries. This fact shows that, under the appropriate conditions, disease fighting and repair processes in the body can be very powerful.

Spontaneous healing is rare and unpredictable, but there are enough well-documented examples of individuals quickly and permanently recovering from 'terminal' and 'uncurable' conditions to stimulate research into how this can happen. Some medical researchers are attempting to induce spontaneous remissions 'on demand', by triggering the body's own defenses against cancer. While there are few answers, it does appear that: 'all the circuitry and machinery is there; the problem is simply to discover how to turn on the right switches to activate the process' (Weil 1995). I have personally seen enough instances of both conventional and complementary practitioners 'turning the right switches' or 'jump-starting the healing process' to know that an understanding of 'spontaneous' healing may not be as far away as we might think. Modern research, complemented by the observations of energy therapists, is teaching us about where to look for the 'circuits' and the 'switches'.

Just as exciting as 'spontaneous' healing is the work on the healing of emotional trauma and abuse. Those who suffer from such afflictions can be just as debilitated as those who have a chronic disease or physical injury. To free a life from emotional pain and agony can be immensely rewarding (see Chs 8 and 11).

The confusion and hostility surrounding energy therapies has contributed significantly to our current medical crisis and the division between so-called conventional and complementary therapies. In the past, the most remarkable success stories of complementary therapists (as well as healings in the religious context) were often dismissed because there was no logical explanation. The practitioners themselves usually could add little in the way of clarification. By bringing recent science into the picture, we are finding the missing links in our images of the human body in health and disease.

References

Brennan BA 1987 Hands of light. A guide to healing through the human energy field. Bantam Books, Toronto

Collinge W 1998 Subtle energy. Where ancient wisdom and modern science meet. Warner Books, New York

Egidio G 1997 Whose hands are these? A gifted healer's miraculous true story. Warner Books, New York

Gauguelin M 1974 The cosmic clocks. Avon Books, New York

Motz J 1998 Hands of life: from the operating room to your home, an energy healer reveals the secrets of using your body's own energy medicine for healing, recovery, and transformation. Bantam Books, New York

Oz M 1998 Healing from the heart: a leading heart surgeon explores the power of complementary medicine. Dutton, New York

Weil A 1995 Spontaneous healing: how to discover and enhance your body's natural ability to maintain and heal itself. Alfred A. Knopf, New York

1 Historical background

In every culture and in every medical tradition before ours, healing was accomplished by moving energy.
Albert Szent-Györgyi (1960)

Energy fields in medicine

The earliest recorded use of electricity for healing dates from 2750 BC, when sick people were exposed to the shocks produced by electric eels (Kellaway 1946). Around 400 BC, Thales rubbed amber and obtained static electricity.

Different forms of magnet healing may be even older. An African mine over 100 000 years old was a source of red iron ore, called bloodstone or ocher, that has been used since ancient times for healing and ceremonial purposes. Magnetite or lodestone was used for healing by the ancient Egyptians, the Chinese, and, later, by the Greeks (Payne 1990).

Various healings are described in the Bible and in other spiritual texts from around the world. The 'laying on of hands' method practiced by Jesus (Fig. 1.1) continues today in some churches and cathedrals. Modern versions of this technique are called 'therapeutic touch', 'healing touch', 'Reiki', or 'polarity therapy', and have become established in many nursing schools and hospitals (e.g. Quinn & Strelkauskas 1993; Quinn 1984, 1992; Krieger 1975). All of these methods are considered energy therapies (see Ch. 6 for discussion of the mechanisms involved).

In 1773, Franz Anton Mesmer (Fig. 1.2A) began using magnets for healing. His patients frequently noticed 'unusual currents' coursing through their bodies prior to the onset of a 'healing crisis' that led to a cure. Soon Mesmer discovered that he could produce the same phenomena without the magnets, simply by passing his hands above the patient's body (Fig. 1.2B). After some careful experimentation, in 1779 Mesmer published his *Memoir on the Discovery of Animal*

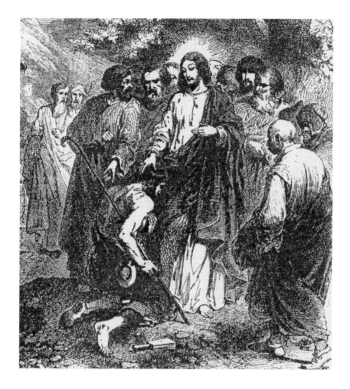

Fig. 1.1 Woodcut from an old bible, showing Jesus healing a leper.

Magnetism (Mesmer 1948). Mesmer felt a sort of attraction and repulsion phenomenon around the body, similar to the sensations one has in handling iron magnets.

Mesmer invited scientists to witness his very popular work with 'incurable' cases, but the scientific and medical community responded mainly with ridicule, animosity, malicious rumours, slander, and fear. It must be said, however, that Mesmer's scientific reputation was not always enhanced by his personal demeanor: 'Clothed in a robe embroidered with Rosicrucian alchemical symbols, he stalked the darkened rooms to the accompaniment of a glass harmonica and actively encouraged his clients to luxuriate in their convulsive crises' (Miller 1995). Three scientific commissions investigated Mesmer's methods, and found his successes to be the result of the imagination of his patients, and not of any real magnetic effect. Benjamin Franklin and Lavoisier were members of the last of these commissions. Franklin considered magnetic

A

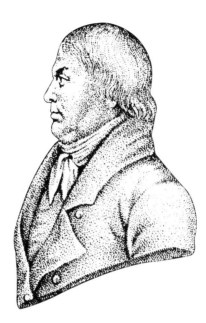

B

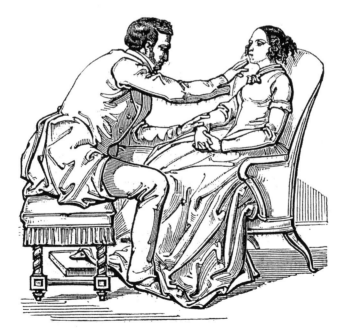

Fig. 1.2 **A** A portrait of Friedrich Anton Mesmer from his 1814 work *Mesmerismus* (Mesmer 1966). **B** A commom Mesmeric posture (from Dupotet 1862, reproduced in Winter 1998), with the 'magnetizer' moving his hand closely over his patient.

emanations 'philosophically unacceptable,' although at the same time he was convinced that electricity was a 'weightless fluid,' and Lavoisier assumed that heat was another one.

Mesmer's method resembled the laying on of hands used by Jesus and other religious figures. Modern methods resembling that of Mesmer include therapeutic touch, polarity therapy, Reiki, aura balancing, and many others. A variety of clinical trials have shown the efficacy of these methods, and, as we shall soon see, research has begun to explain how they are effective.

An emotional controversy

Since ancient times, people have had a deep fear of the powerful and invisible forces of nature. Shamans and other religious figures derived authority from their ability to 'explain' the unknown, predict celestial events, and calm the people (Calvin 1991). In many respects, science is another way of 'seeing' and explaining that which is normally hidden from our view. For biologists, the relationship between energy fields and life has been a subject of bitter and continuous controversy for over 400 years. The battle concerns a fundamental disagreement about the nature of life. Competing philosophies have generated much emotion and dogma. The argument is referred to as mechanism vs vitalism.

Mechanism vs vitalism

Mechanists hold that life obeys the laws of chemistry and physics, and will ultimately be totally explained by those laws. In contrast, vitalists have historically held to the belief that life will never be explained by normal physics and chemistry, and that there is some kind of mysterious 'life force' that is separate from the known laws of nature and that distinguishes living from non-living matter. This concept is ancient and universal, appearing in some form or another in many different cultures and religions.

With the discovery of electricity, some vitalists associated electrical fields with a life force (for a detailed account of the history of this subject, see Becker & Marino 1982).

Early electrotherapy

Medical electricity had its golden era between the late 1700s and the early 1900s. During that period, a variety of electrical healing devices were developed and were widely used by physicians for treating a range of ailments (Geddes 1984).

Four different forms of electricity were used:

◆ Static, or franklinic electricity

◆ Direct, or galvanic current

◆ Induction-coil, or faradic current

◆ High-frequency, or d'Arsonval current.

Clinical electrotherapy was thriving at the same time that vitalism was being rejected by mainstream science. By 1884 it was estimated that 10 000 physicians in the USA were using electricity every day for therapeutic purposes, totally without the blessing of science. Figure 1.3 shows an electromagnetic healing device patented by Elias Smith in 1869, and Figure 1.4 shows a French version (d'Arsonval 1894).

A popular approach was the 'electric hand' shown in Figure 1.5. The patient sat on a stool with his bare feet on a metal plate connected to an induction coil. An electrode attached to the other terminal of the coil was held in one hand by the therapist. The therapist's other hand – the 'electric hand' – was used to stroke or massage the patient over various parts of the body (Ziemssen 1864). For many, a 'general faradization' of the whole body produced an ecstatic experience. 'Localized faradization' of specific regions was used to treat a variety of medical problems. In some cases, special electrodes were used to

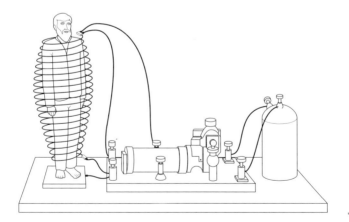

Fig. 1.3 Healing device patented by E. Smith on October 19, 1869, US Patent No. 96,044. For convenience the coil is in two parts so the patient can step into the lower one and have the upper one placed over the head. Current flowing through the coil creates a magnetic field around and through the body. This is augmented by passing another current through the body from the head to the feet.

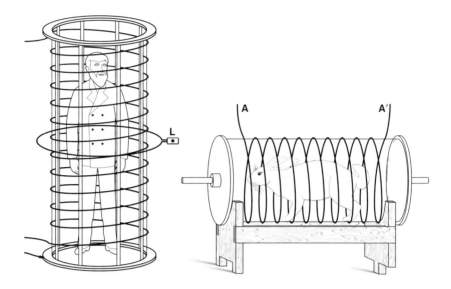

Fig. 1.4 French version of the Smith invention, described by d'Arsonval (1894).

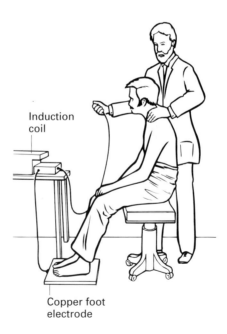

Induction coil

Copper foot electrode

Fig. 1.5 The 'electric hand' method widely used in the late 1800s. The therapist and patient are connected in series to an induction coil that generates electricity. Here the therapist is shown massaging and 'faradizing' the patient's shoulder with his left hand.

stimulate particular parts of the body. It was claimed that nearly all diseases could be cured by electricity, provided it could be passed through the blood.

One discovery made using the electric hand was that stimulation of specific points on the body surface causes the underlying muscles to contract. In 1864, Ziemssen charted the locations of these points, which are now called 'muscle points' or 'motor points' (Basmajian 1979). Using fresh cadavers, Ziemssen marked many of the motor points, dissected the underlying tissue, and found they were the places where the nerves entered the muscles. Subsequently, in 1867 Duchenne (1959) published his classic studies of the muscle points (Fig. 1.6) that gave rise to the modern field of medical electromyography, in which electrical recordings are made of the activity of the motor points to determine whether the muscle is properly innervated.

The discoveries of the cellular and molecular basis of life, the bacterial origin of infectious diseases, Darwin's theory of evolution, and the electrical aspects of

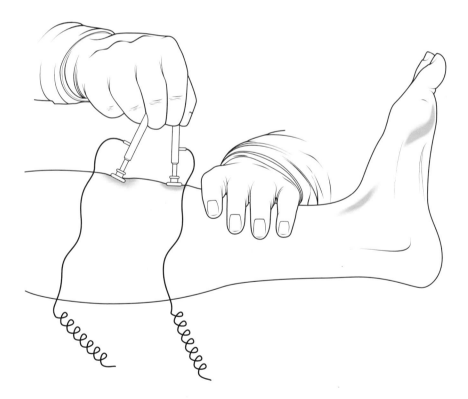

Fig. 1.6 Duchenne's (1867) illustration of electrical stimulation of muscles (Duchenne 1959). His research founded the modern medical field of electromyography.

nerve conduction were all taken by the scientific establishment as the final blows to the vitalist position. All of life, from its beginnings in the primordial sea to its present level of complexity, could be explained scientifically. Organisms, like machines, could be broken down into their components and studied piece by piece until all mysteries could be solved. It was just a matter of time and hard work before everything about life and disease could be understood. For the vitalist position, fundamental discoveries in biology caused a steady retreat, but the basic mystery of the driving force for nature remained.

Edwin D. Babbitt

In 1873, Edwin D. Babbitt (Fig. 1.7A), a minister in East Orange, New Jersey, published his classic treatise *The Principles of Light and Color* (Babbitt 1873, 1967, 1992). He had secluded himself in a darkened room for several weeks, and, when he emerged, he discovered he had acquired a greatly heightened visual sensitivity and could see energy fields around human bodies. Some would dismiss this as some form of hallucination, were it not for his beautiful etchings showing the fields around the head (Fig. 1.7B). A century later, we know that the field Babbitt observed corresponds to that expected from neuro-currents flowing through the interhemispheric fibers of the corpus callosum (Fig. 1.7C).

A

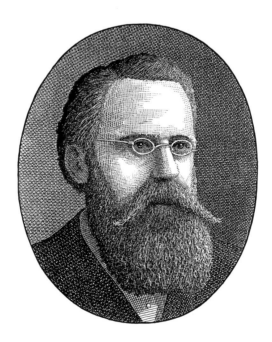

B

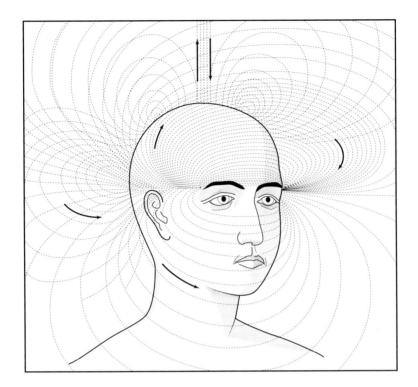

C

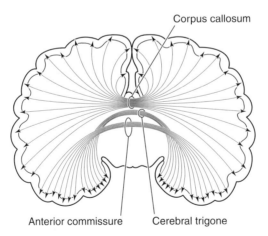

Corpus callosum

Anterior commissure   Cerebral trigone

Fig. 1.7 A A portrait of Edwin D. Babbitt, MD, LLD, from his 1873 work *The Principles of Light and Color* (Babbitt 1873, 1967, 1992). **B** The 'magnetic curves' as drawn by Babbitt in *The Principles of Light and Color* (Babbitt 1873, 1967, 1992) (reproduced with permission of Sun Publishing). **C** The interhemispheric fibers (Pansky 1975) (Reproduced with kind permission of Macmillan).

Babbitt applied various colors in therapy. He taught his methods to others, and had a wide following.

Electrotherapy at the turn of the 20th century

By 1900, a wide variety of electrical and magnetic healing devices were on the market, providing therapies for every disease and problem. Figure 1.8 illustrates some items listed in the 1902 catalogue from Sears Roebuck in Chicago, Illinois. Many claims were made about the miraculous healing powers of these products. Electric belts, bands, chains, plasters, and garters were 'capable of providing a quick cure of all nervous and organic disorders arising from any cause' and Dr Hammond's Nerve and Brain Pills were 'positively guaranteed to cure any disease'.

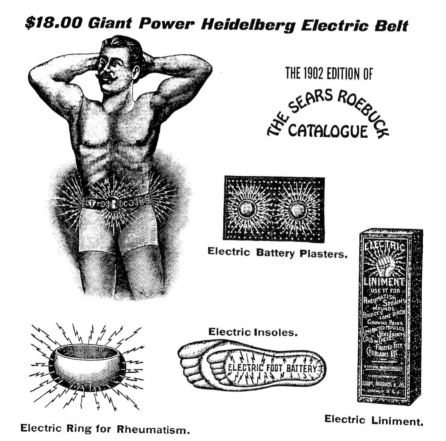

Fig. 1.8 Electrical healing devices listed in the 1902 Catalogue of the Sears Roebuck Company, Chicago, Illinois.

There was virtually no systematic verification that any of these devices had therapeutic value. Note that we are not saying these products were ineffective, but that there simply was no scientific evidence one way or the other.

Flexner report

The total absence of standards for medical education and clinical practice in the USA led to the passage of the federal Pure Food and Drugs Act of 1906, and to the publication in 1910 of the Flexner report. The latter established science as the basis for medicine and clinical education. Medical schools were completely overhauled. Electrotherapy was declared scientifically unsupportable and was legally excluded from clinical practice. Many doctors had equipment removed from their offices and taken to 'museums of quackery'. They were told that if they wanted to continue using electrotherapies, they would be doing it in prison! Dr Hammond's pills were no longer sold through the Sears Catalogue.

The 20th Century

Electrobiology

In the meantime, rapid progress began to take place in electrobiology – the study of the electrical properties of living systems. Various useful diagnostic tools were developed that involved recording the electrical fields produced by organs such as the heart, the other muscles, the eyes, and the brain (some of this is explored further in Ch. 2).

With progress in electrobiology, electricity gradually lost its mystery and became less attractive as the elusive force the vitalists were searching for. This does not mean that vitalism is dead, nor does it mean we fully understand all of the energies and forces of nature, including electricity and magnetism, and their roles in living systems.

The emotional and dogmatic fervour of the past persists. There continues to be a strong academic bias against any suggestion that the electrical and magnetic fields generated by tissues and organs might have any important biological purpose – they are widely thought to be mere by-products of cellular activities, useful for diagnosis only. We shall see, though, that this view is no longer accurate. Biological fields are not just by-products of physiological processes, they are part of the mechanism by which the body communicates with itself. Research on this topic is underway in medical and academic research centres around the world. 'Electromagnetic medicine' is beginning to revive, but with far more sophisticated science to support it.

In the climate produced by the Flexner report, some prominent scientists, seeking to explore the possible role of electricity in the control of growth and development, realized they were entering politically hazardous territory. Some researchers obtained academic tenure by doing mainstream research before they began investigating fields. In this way they could be free to explore the role of energy fields in living processes without the danger of being fired from their university positions.

Harold Saxton Burr

One pioneer was Harold Saxton Burr (Fig. 1.9), who obtained his PhD degree at Yale in 1915 and became a full professor at Yale School of Medicine in 1929. He was appointed E. K. Hunt Professor of Anatomy in 1933 and remained in the post for 40 years. His early work was on the development of the nervous system, and he published nearly 20 papers on this subject between 1916 and 1935.

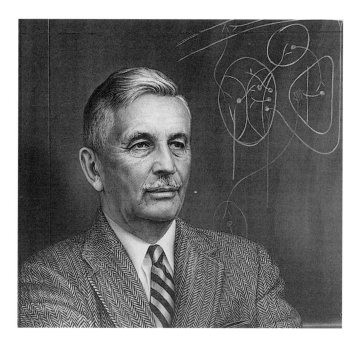

Fig. 1.9 Harold Saxton Burr. From a painting by Artzybasheff presented to the Yale University School of Medicine on December 6, 1957 by the Burr Portrait Committee on behalf of Dr Burr's colleagues and former students. (Reproduced by courtesy of the Yale Art Gallery and the Yale University School of Medicine.)

In 1932, Burr began a series of important and controversial studies of the role of electricity in development and disease. From his work on the development of the nervous system, Burr realized how little was actually known about the control of form in animals. Molecular genetics was revealing how the parts of the body are manufactured, but there was little understanding of the 'blueprint' that directs their assembly into the whole organism. While there is widespread enthusiasm about the discoveries being made in molecular biology, the mystery of the 'blueprint' continues to this day.

Burr had many students and collaborators, some of whom were, or became, leading figures in science. In all, he published some 93 papers, and stimulated his colleagues in the production of about 100 more. He also wrote a book about his conclusions entitled *Blueprint for Immortality: the Electric Patterns of Life* (Burr 1972), which was also published under the title *The Fields of Life*.

Burr's work on energy fields from 1932 to 1956 was way out of step with the mainstream medicine and biology of the time. This was a period of explosive growth in pharmaceutical medicine and in the use of X-rays for diagnosis. Antibiotics were winning the war against disease, and the thrust of medical research and public policy was toward 'a pill for every problem'. The public was dazzled by the seemingly continuous and accelerating rate of scientific and medical progress. There was a very successful concept of bioenergetics, but it was entirely confined to the study of biochemical reactions and the ways molecules store and release metabolic energy.

In the 1950s, a visitor to Burr's ancestral home, Mansewood, in Lyme, Connecticut, would discover various kinds of trees connected to recording voltmeters: Burr was convinced that all living things, from mice to humans, from seeds to trees, are formed and controlled by fields that can be measured with standard detectors. He published a series of articles on how the electric fields of trees change in advance of weather patterns and other atmospheric phenomena. Burr was convinced that the 'fields of life' are the basic blueprints for all living things; the fields reflect physical and mental conditions, and are therefore useful for diagnostic purposes.

During the period when Burr was researching energy fields, most biologists and physicians were certain that all notions of energy therapy and 'life force' were complete nonsense. The experiences of practitioners and patients of energy therapies were dismissed, either by ignoring them, or by stating that the patients were victims of deception, illusion, trickery, fakery, quackery, hallucination, or the placebo effect. Scientists could say with certainty that any energy field around an organism would be far too weak to be detected. If such a field existed, it surely had no biological significance. Healing with energy fields was fantasy, and any notion that light could be emitted by the body was certainly quite foolish.

As a student of the history of medicine, Burr was well aware that work published ahead of its time remains in the libraries and is available to future generations when its moment arrives. Such a period is upon us, and Burr's articles are highly recommended, both for the serious student of energetic bodywork and/or movement therapy and for biomedical researchers exploring the role of energy fields in health and disease. A complete listing of Burr's articles can be found in the *Yale Journal of Biology and Medicine* (Burr 1957) and at the end of Burr's own book (Burr 1972).

In retrospect, Burr's discoveries anticipated many of the breakthroughs that are being made around the world at the present time. His published work, and that of Robert O. Becker (Becker & Selden 1985, Becker 1990) are excellent introductions to the subject. The remainder of this book will provide modern scientific perspective on the 'life force' and 'healing energy'.

Fields in diagnosis

The use of fields for diagnosis is based on the premise that every physiological process in the body has an electrical counterpart. Burr reiterated a position taken years earlier by the physiologist A. P. Mathews: 'Every excess of action, every change in the physical state of the protoplasm of any organ, or any area in the embryo or in the egg, produces, it is believed, an electrical disturbance' (Mathews 1903).

As we shall soon see, modern research has confirmed the observations of Mathews and Burr. Not only does every event in the body, either normal or pathological, produce electrical changes, it also produces alterations of the magnetic fields in the spaces around the body. Recent research describes how this comes about; valuable summaries have been published by Brewitt (1996, 1999).

Ovulation as an example

In 1935 Burr described the detection of ovulation by monitoring the substantial voltage changes during the ovulation cycle. Others attempted to repeat Burr's work, but their results were not consistent. Burr continued to refine his approach, and reported in 1936 and 1938 that the timing of ovulation in women could be determined by daily measurements of the electric field between one finger from each hand. This was confirmed by another scientist in 1939, but others continued to have inconsistent results. Burr continued to investigate the problem, publishing his last paper on the subject in 1953.

By 1974 the causes of variation in the ovulation potentials had been determined, and a fertility control system based on Burr's work was awarded a US patent (Friedenberg et al 1975). The patent is interesting reading because it documents the reason for the inconsistency of previous studies. The ovulation cycle is but one of many bodily rhythms that produce an oscillating electric field. Detection of the ovulation cycle requires careful filtering, to eliminate interference from other electrical rhythms generated by the other organs in the body, such as the heart and brain (see Fig. 1.10). Once the electrical rhythms from other organs have been removed by filtration, the monthly rhythm of the ovary can be recorded (Fig. 1.11).

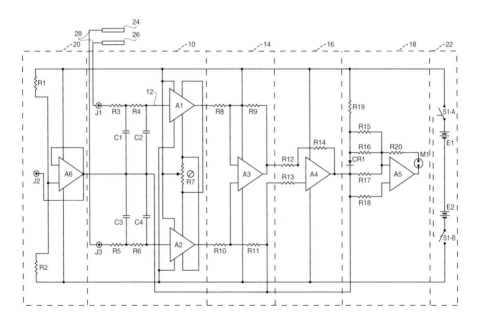

Fig. 1.10 The circuit patented by Friedenberg, Reese & Reading (1975) to separate the monthly electrical rhythm of the ovary from the rhythms of other organs in the body. The patent describes this as 'the combined circuitry for milli-volt measurement including the critical means of high impedance and high common mode rejection combined with sufficient isolation and filtration of the essential circuit to reliably indicate and measure the low D.C. ovulation potential'. From US Patent 3,924.609.

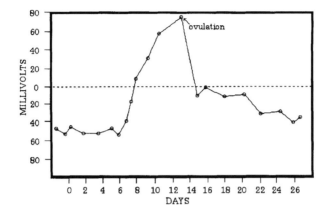

Fig. 1.11 The electrical rhythm of the ovulation cycle in the human female as recorded between a finger from each hand. Before and after ovulation the potentials are negative. About 5–6 days before ovulation, the potential begins to rise and increases above zero a few days before ovulation. Afterwards there is a rapid decline to below zero, at which time the body is free of a fertilizable ovum. The curve is taken from US Patent 3,924.609.

Early cancer detection

Another controversial area of investigation concerned the detection of cancer. Burr was convinced that diseases would show up in the energy field before symptoms of pathology, such as tumors. His theory was that if the disturbed energy field could be detected and restored to normal, the pathology could be prevented. This is obviously a concept with profound medical significance.

In 1936, Burr and his colleagues began a series of studies on the relation between electrical fields and cancer, beginning with spontaneous mammary tumors in mice. Large voltage changes were detected with electrodes attached to the chest from 10 days to 2 weeks before the tumors appeared. In 1945, British researchers attempted to repeat Burr's experiments, but without success. Burr continued to work on the problem, and published his last cancer paper in 1949. The following year, critiques of Burr's work were summarized by Crane (1950).

Confirmation of Burr's cancer research

Some of the most important research on the role of energy fields in health and disease has come from research based on the theory and practice of acupuncture. Sadly, this work has been largely ignored by biomedical researchers because of skepticism about the existence of the acupuncture meridians and points. In this unfortunate way valuable insights about energetics have long been excluded from mainstream medical thinking. This situation is rapidly changing.

In the late 1940s, while Burr was winding down his cancer research, Reinhold Voll in Germany was testing the electrical resistance of acupuncture pathways and correlating the conductances with specific pathological problems. He suggested that inflammation increases conductances, while organ degeneration and tissue necrosis decreases them. A weakness of Voll's papers in English (Voll 1980, 1989) was that he focused on his patient's conditions rather than on the actual conductance data. Voll's collaborator, Schimmel, published the conductance data documenting Voll's conclusions (see Tiller 1988).

In 1973, two British clinicians working at a tuberculosis sanitarium showed that the conductance at the acupuncture point Liver 8, located on the knee, was about 18 times higher in patients with known liver disease (cirrhosis or acute hepatitis) compared to patients with no liver disease (Bergsmann & Woolley-Hart 1973). Of course a phenomenon such as this, no matter how robust and reliable and repeatable, has little meaning to the Western biomedical researcher, to whom it is obvious that liver problems reside in the liver, and have nothing whatsoever to do with the knee. Oriental medicine, in contrast, considers that the function, Liver, does not reside in a particular place in the body (the organ that Western medicine refers to as the liver). Instead, Liver is viewed as a function that exists throughout the organism, and that can be treated at a wide variety of points a distance away from the physical structure called 'liver'. There are now very good reasons for taking a closer look at the Oriental medical perspective, as we shall soon see.

In 1985, Sullivan and colleagues reported that patients with lung disease (confirmed by chest X-rays) had 30% lower electrical conductances at lung points. Other research, summarized by Brewitt (1996, 1999), showed the cellular basis for these effects. Specifically, viral and bacterial infections, as well as cancer, affect the ionic and water content and pH of the extracellular fluids, and thereby affect the cell membrane potentials and tissue conductances.

More detailed study (Surowiec et al 1987) showed that the conductance changes in tumors are highly frequency dependent. Direct measurements showed 6.0–7.5 times higher conductances in tumors compared to normal tissues (Smith et al 1986). In later stages of both cancer and AIDS, tissues begin to deteriorate and electrical conductances drop.

In 1996, Brewitt re-analyzed some of Burr's original data using modern statistical methods. There is no question that Burr was correct: disease states can be detected by measuring changes in the electrical conductances of tissues, making possible early diagnosis and treatments.

In 1994, Weiss et al reported that skin surface electrical potentials can be used for the differential diagnosis of breast lesions. The electrical changes arise because rapidly proliferating and transformed cells have lower membrane potentials compared with normal cells (Binggeli & Weinstein 1986). This has been demonstrated for tumor cells from both breast (Marino et al 1994) and colon (Davies et al 1987, Goller et al 1986). The altered membrane potentials extend from the cancerous area to the skin surface above the lesion. The correlation between cell membrane potentials and cell proliferation was detailed in a classic paper by Cone (1970). Cuzick and colleagues (Cuzick et al 1998, Cuzick 1998) have reported clinical trials of a method for detecting breast cancer using skin electropotential measurements. This non-invasive method is important because it offers the opportunity to resolve the uncertainty of lump detection, whether by self-palpation or by mammograms. In most cases, lumps are benign, but the methods needed to prove this in an individual case are invasive. Burr's goal of a non-invasive and risk-free test for the presence of cancer is being realized.

Conclusion

While the old emotional and dogmatic biases persist, the trend of modern research is toward explaining and validating the experiences of practitioners and recipients of energy therapies, including the type of healing that takes place in the religious context. Vitalism, as an undiscovered 'life force', has not been ruled out, and the role of spirit is not to be discounted. However, much is being discovered about how electricity, magnetism, and other energy fields are created and utilized by living organisms.

Harold Saxton Burr's methods did not become part of accepted clinical practice during his lifetime, but his reasoning was sound. Another example of modern work confirming Burr's concepts comes from a study undertaken in Rome which explored the biomagnetic fields produced near the head during epileptic seizures. In some cases the epilepsy was caused by tumors that did not show up in electroencephalogram (EEG)s or computer-aided tomography (CAT) scans, but that could be detected by biomagnetic recordings (Modena et al 1982). Similarly, magnetoencephalography is being used to improve the accuracy of functional magnetic resonance imaging (MRI) brain mapping (Beisteiner et al 1997).

For Burr, the link between biology and physics was not mysterious, or unfathomable, or subtle. The energies so thoroughly studied by physicists surround, and penetrate, and are produced by all living things. Biological electricity, for example, is no different from any other kind of electricity, nor does it obey different laws.

As a phenomenon, bioenergy fields have gone from scientific 'nonsense' to an important and expanding subject of biomedical research. In later chapters we see not only that fields can be detected a distance from the body, but also that scientists are explaining how these fields are generated, why they become distorted when pathology is present, why living systems are so extraordinarily sensitive to fields, and how fields can be used in healing.

The information that is emerging has direct relevance to all clinical methods. Documenting the fascinating tale of how our outlook is changing is the goal of this book.

References

Babbitt E D 1873 The principles of light and color. College of Fine Forces, East Orange, NJ

Babbitt E D 1967 The principles of light and color. Citadel Press, Secaucus, NH (repr. of 1st edn of 1873)

Babbitt E D 1992 The principles of light and color. Sun Publishing, Santa Fe, NM (repr. of 1st edn of 1873)

Basmajian J V 1979 Muscles alive: their functions revealed by electromyography. Williams & Wilkins, Baltimore

Becker R O 1990 Cross currents: the perils of electropollution, the promise of electromedicine. Jeremy P. Tarcher, Los Angeles

Becker R O, Marino A A 1982 Electromagnetism and life. State University of New York Press, Albany

Becker R O, Selden G 1985 The body electric: electromagnetism and the foundation of life. William Morrow, New York

Beisteiner R, Erdler M, Teichtmeister C et al 1997 Magnetoencephalography may help to improve functional MRI brain mapping. European Journal of Neuroscience 9(5):1072–1077

Bergsmann O, Woolley-Hart A 1973 Differences in electrical skin conductivity between acupuncture points and adjacent skin areas. American Journal of Acupuncture 1:27–32

Binggeli R, Weinstein R C 1986 Membrane potentials and sodium channels: hypotheses for growth regulation and cancer formation based on changes in sodium channels and gap junctions. Journal of Theoretical Biology 123:377–401

Brewitt B 1996 Quantitative analysis of electrical skin conductance in diagnosis: historical and current views of bioelectric medicine. Journal of Naturopathic Medicine 6(1):66–75

Brewitt B 1999 Electromagnetic medicine and HIV/AIDS treatment: clinical data and hypothesis for mechanism of action. In: Standish L J, Calabrese C, Galatino M L (eds) AIDS and alternative medicine: the current state of the science. Harcourt Brace, New York

Burr H S 1957 Harold Saxton Burr. Yale Journal of Biology and Medicine 30(3):161–167

Burr H S 1972 Blueprint for immortality. CW Daniel, Saffron Walden

Calvin W H 1991 How the shaman stole the moon: in search of ancient prophet-scientists from Stonehenge to the Grand Canyon. Bantam Books, New York

Cone C D Jr 1970 Variation of the transmembrane potential level as a basic mechanism of mitosis control. Oncogenesis 24:438–470

Crane E E 1950 Bioelectric potentials, their maintenance and function. Progress in Biophysics and Biophysical Chemistry 1:85–136

Cuzick J 1998 Continuation of the international breast cancer intervention study (IBIS). European Journal of Cancer 34(11):1647–1648

Cuzick J R, Holland V, Barth R et al 1998 Electropotential measurements as a new diagnostic modality for breast cancer. Lancet 352:359–363

d'Arsonval J-A 1894 Action de l'électricité sur les êtres vivants. Cours d'Appel, Paris

Davies R J, Weidema WF, Sandle G I, Palmer L, Deschner EE, DeCosse J J 1987 Sodium transport in a mouse model of colonic carcinogenesis. Cancer Research 47:4646–4650

Duchenne G B A (1959) (trans. E B Kaplan 1949 from 1st edn 1867) Physiologie des mouvements. W B Saunders, Philadelphia

Dupotet C 1862 L'art du magnétiseur. Paris

Friedenberg R, Reese W, Reading W H 1975 Detector device and process for detecting ovulation. United States Patent 3,924.609. December 9, 1975

Geddes L A 1984 A short history of the electrical stimulation of excitable tissue including electrotherapeutic applications. Physiologist 27(1):S1–S47

Goller D A, Weidema W F, Davies R J 1986 Transmural electrical potential difference as an early marker in colon cancer. Archives of Surgery 121:345–350

Kellaway P 1946 The part played by electric fish in the early history of bioelectricity and electrotherapy. Bulletin of the History of Medicine 20:112–132

Krieger D 1975 Therapeutic touch: the imprimatur of nursing. American Journal of Nursing 5:784–787

Marino A A, Ilev I G, Schwalke M A et al 1994 Association between cell membrane potential and breast cancer. Tumor Biology 15:82–89

Mathews A P 1903 Electric polarity in hydroids. American Journal of Physiology 8:294–299

Mesmer A 1948 Mesmerism: with an introduction by Gilbert Frankau. Macdonald, London [This is Mesmer's Memoir of 1779.]

Mesmer F A 1966 Mesmerismus: oder System der Wechselwirkungen, Theorie und Anwendung des thierischen Magnetismus als die allgemeine Heilkunde zur Erhaltung des Menschen. Translated by Karl Christian Wolfart. E. J. Bonset, Amsterdam [Mesmer's work was first published in 1814]

Miller J 1995 Going unconscious. In: Silvers RB (ed) Hidden histories of science. Granta Books, London, pp 1–35

Modena I, Ricci G B, Barbanera S, Leoni R, Romani G L. Carelli P 1982 Biomagnetic measurements of spontaneous brain activity in epileptic patients. Electroencephalography and Clinical Neurophysiology 54:622–628

Pansky B 1975 Dynamic anatomy and physiology. Macmillan, New York, fig 8.7, p 253

Payne B 1990 The body magnetic. Privately published, Santa Cruz, C A

Quinn J F 1984 Therapeutic touch as energy exchange: testing the theory. Advances in Nursing Science 6:42–49

Quinn J F 1992 The senior's therapeutic touch education program. Holistic Nurse Practitioner 7:32–37

Quinn J F, Strelkauskas A J 1993 Psychoimmunologic effects of therapeutic touch on practitioners and recently bereaved recipients: a pilot study. Advances in Nursing Science 15(4):13–26

Smith S R, Foster K R, Wolf G L 1986 Dielectric properties of VX-2 carcinoma versus normal liver tissue. IEEE Transactions of Biomedical Engineering BME 33:522–524

Sullivan S G, Eggleston W W, Martinoff J T, Kroenig RJ 1985 Evoked electrical conductivity on the lung acupuncture points in healthy individuals and confirmed lung cancer patients. American Journal of Acupuncture 13(3) 261–266

Surowiec A J, Stuchly S S, Keaney M, Swarup A 1987 Dielectric polarization of animal lung at radio frequencies. IEEE Transactions of Biomedical Engineering BME 34:62–66

Szent-Györgyi A 1960 Introduction to a submolecular biology. Academic Press, New York

Tiller W A 1988 On the evolution of electrodermal diagnostic instruments. Journal of Advancement in Medicine 1:41–56

Weiss B A, Ganepola A P, Freeman H P, Hsu Yu-S, Faupel M L 1994 Surface electrical potentials as a new modality in the diagnosis of breast lesions: a preliminary report. Breast Disease 7:91–98

Voll R 1980 The phenomenon of medicine testing in electro-acupuncture according to Voll. American Journal of Acupuncture 8:97–104

Voll R 1989 Twenty years of electroacupuncture diagnosis in Germany: a progress report. American Journal of Acupuncture (Special EAV edition):5–14

Winter A 1998 Mesmerized: powers of mind in Victorian Britain. University of Chicago Press, Chicago, fig 1, p 2

Ziemssen H 1864 Die Electricitat in der Medicin, 2nd edn. Von August Hirschwald, Berlin

2 Measuring the fields of life

Something deeply hidden has to be behind things.
Albert Einstein (while playing with a compass his father had given him)

In the current era of rapid scientific progress, many of the concepts we were absolutely certain about 20 years ago are no longer true at all. But of all the tales of exploration and discovery that could be told, none is more fascinating than the story of the human energy field. In a few decades scientists have gone from a conviction that there is no such thing as energy fields in and around the human body to an absolute certainty that they exist. Consequently, practitioners of traditional energy methods are beginning to be investigated by biomedical researchers. The resulting synthesis benefits everyone, particularly those who have injuries or diseases that are difficult to treat with other techniques.

Medical interest has focused on the *magnetic* fields around the body, which are now referred to as *biomagnetic* fields. Interest in biomagnetism has spread widely in the biomedical research community. The role of other fields, including electricity, light, heat, gravity, kinetic energy, and sound, will be taken up in later chapters.

Heart electricity

Our story begins with the investigation of bioelectricity, for it is from electric currents that magnetic fields arise. If you are not a physicist or an electrical engineer, and do not understand electricity and magnetism, you have excellent company. For example, we recognize different forms of energy, such as electricity, magnetism, heat, light, electromagnetism, kinetic energy of motion, sound, gravity, vibration, elastic energy, etc. But there must be some fundamental principle that underlies these different forms of energy.

Albert Einstein spent the last decades of his life in an unsuccessful search for a 'common denominator,' or the 'something deeply hidden' that has to be behind the various forms of energy. At a fundamental level, we still do not know exactly what electricity and magnetism really are. The electron is a basic unit, and has properties such as charge, mass, and gravity, but a deeper explanation of how these properties arise is missing. Valuable perspectives on this problem have been published by Day (1989, 1996) and Wolff (1993, 1997).

Around the turn of the 20th century, a Dutch physician, Willem Einthoven, discovered that heart electricity could be routinely recorded with a very sensitive galvanometer (Einthoven 1906). Einthoven received a Nobel Prize in 1924 for this discovery. His method has been improved to the point that the electrocardiogram is a standard tool for medical diagnosis.

We now know that each heartbeat begins with a pulse of electricity through the heart muscle. This electricity arises because a large number of charged particles (ions of sodium, potassium, chloride, calcium, and magnesium) flow across the muscle membranes to excite contraction. These currents also spread out into surrounding tissues.

Some of the flow of electricity from the heart is through the circulatory system, which is an excellent conductor of electricity because of its high salt content. As the circulation carries blood to every tissue, heart electricity flows everywhere in the body. Hence the electrocardiogram can be picked up anywhere on the skin, even from the toes. Cardiologists know that if there is a problem in the functioning of part of the heart, the electrocardiogram will be distorted in a characteristic manner. The enigma is that most cardiologists are certain that the heart's electrical field is a by-product, almost a waste product, of the heart's activities, and has no significant physiological role except as a diagnostic tool.

Magnetism from electricity

It is a basic law in physics that when an electric current flows through a conductor, a magnetic field is created in the surrounding space. This phenomenon was discovered by accident by Hans Christian Oersted during a physics lecture he was giving in Copenhagen in 1820.

Heart magnetism

On the basis of Oersted's discovery, some scientists predicted that the heart's electricity should create heart magnetism, but it was not until 1963 that anyone was able to detect it in the laboratory. In that year, Gerhard Baule and Richard McFee (1963), at the electrical engineering department of Syracuse University in New York, used a pair of 2 million-turn coils on the chest to pick up the magnetic field produced by the electrical activity of the heart muscle (Fig. 2.1). The heart was chosen for study because it produces the strongest electrical and magnetic activity of any tissue in the body. (The fact that the functioning heart produces a strong pulsating magnetic field, spreading out in front of and behind the body, is important in itself, and is discussed in more detail later.)

One of the academic questions created by the discovery of the heart's magnetic field is the location of the boundary between the organism and the environment. In the past, we could define an individual as that which lies within the skin; but it is a fact of physics that energy fields are unbounded. The biomagnetic field of the heart extends indefinitely into space. While its strength diminishes with distance, there is no point at which we can say the field ends. In practice, the field gets weaker and weaker until it becomes undetectable in the noise produced by other fields in the environment; but scientists are constantly developing tricks to make their instruments more sensitive and to separate signals from noise.

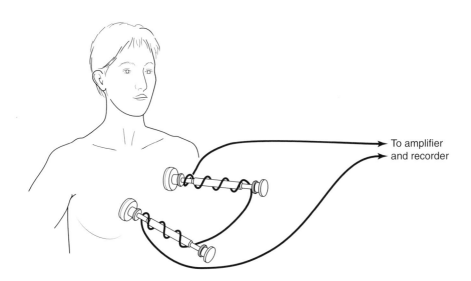

Fig. 2.1 Set-up used to detect the magnetic field of the heart. The two coils each have 2 million turns of wire wound around dumbell-shaped cores of a magnetic material called ferrite. The wires go to an amplifier and recording system. The heart's field is about one-millionth that of the Earth's. (After Baule GM, McFee R 1963 Detection of the magnetic field of the heart. American Heart Journal 66:95–96, with permission.)

A quantum breakthrough

Baule & McFee (1963) predicted that the heart produces magnetic fields, and they went to a lot of trouble to detect those fields. This was a definite breakthrough, but what happened next was far more astonishing. A discovery in quantum physics led to the development of instruments that can map the energy fields of the human body with unprecedented sensitivity and accuracy. For example, there are devices that can pick up the field of the heart 15 feet away from the body.

In the same year as the article by Baule & McFee was published, a number of scientists (Anderson & Rowell 1963, Shapiro 1963) showed that something that seems impossible could actually happen. The seemingly impossible event was the movement of pairs of electrons through a material (called an insulator) that, according to classical physics, the electrons should not be able to penetrate. The phenomenon is called tunneling, and is something that is forbidden in the classical world, the world we are familiar with, but easy in the quantum realm. The reason for this difference is that in the quantum world, classical *particles* such as electrons are at the same time *waves*, and waves can do tricks that solid particles cannot do.

Several kinds of tunneling can take place, and they are called Josephson effects, named after an English physicist, Brian Josephson, who predicted them in 1962 while he was a graduate student at the University of Cambridge (Josephson 1962, 1965; Langenberg et al 1966). In 1973 Josephson received a Nobel Prize for his work.

The SQUID magnetometer

If a thin insulating barrier is placed between two superconductors (such as two metals cooled in liquid helium) a supercurrent consisting of pairs of electrons will flow across the barrier. Josephson effects are utilized in electronic devices and ultra-fast computers. But for us the most exciting application is in the SQUID (an acronym for superconducting quantum interference device). A SQUID consists of one or more Josephson junctions immersed in liquid helium. The device was developed by J. E. Zimmerman and his colleagues (Zimmerman et al 1970, Zimmerman 1972). Under the appropriate conditions, the properties of the Josephson junction become exceedingly sensitive to ambient magnetic fields. Figure 2.2 shows the design of a SQUID magnetometer of the kind used to study biomagnetic fields.

SQUIDs and arrays of SQUIDs are now being used in medical research laboratories around the world to map the biomagnetic fields produced by physio-

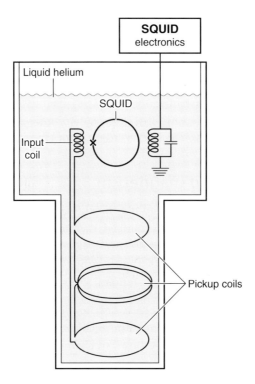

Fig. 2.2 Basic design of the SQUID magnetometer used to detect biomagnetic fields around the human body. The biomagnetic field induces a current flow in the pickup coils. The input coil influences the Josephson junctions in the SQUID proper, and changes in the properties of the junctions are sensed by another circuit that is connected to various amplifiers and filters of the SQUID electronics. The coils and the Josephson junctions are immersed in liquid helium to maintain the superconducting state. (After Kaufman L et al 1984, with kind permission from Annals of the New York Academy of Sciences and Dr Lloyd Kaufman.)

logical processes inside the human body. A global network of SQUIDs is also being used to monitor moment-to-moment fluctuations in the geomagnetic field of the earth.

Magnetocardiography

The first biological application of the SQUID took place inside a heavily shielded room at MIT's Francis Bitter National Magnet Laboratory in Cambridge, Massachusetts. The shielding was essential because the heart's field is one-millionth of the earth's magnetic field and one-thousandth of the varying background magnetic field in an urban environment.

Cohen and his colleagues (Cohen 1967, Cohen et al 1970) described the heart's magnetic field with more clarity and sensitivity than ever before. Their work laid the foundation for a whole new field of diagnostics: magnetocardiography. Figure 2.3 shows a recording of the magnetocardiogram, with a standard electrocardiogram from skin electrodes beside it for comparison.

Brain electricity and magnetism

A few years after Einthoven received his Nobel Prize for the discovery of heart electricity, Hans Berger (1929) announced that much smaller electric fields could also be recorded from the brain, using electrodes attached to the scalp (Fig. 2.5A). With some refinements, the recordings (which came to be known as electroencephalograms) became a standard diagnostic method in neurology, serving as an index of health and disease in the brain.

In 1972, Cohen was able to extend his SQUID measurements to the fields produced by the brain. The set-up is shown in Figure 2.4. The brain fields proved to be hundreds of times weaker than the heart's field, and a lot of tinkering and adjusting and engineering went into re-desiging the SQUID so that it could detect these minute fields. The result was the first ever recording of the biomagnetic field of the brain. Figure 2.5A shows an electroencephalogram (EEG).

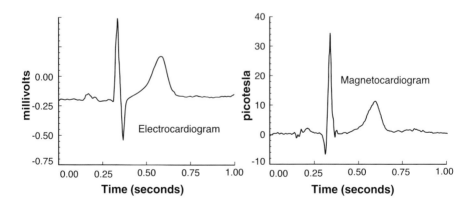

Fig. 2.3 Recordings of the heart's electric field or electrocardiogram (left) and the corresponding magnetic field or magnetocardiogram (right). (After Brockmeier et al 1995, with kind permission from Dr Konrad Brockmeier and Elsevier Science, IOS Press.)

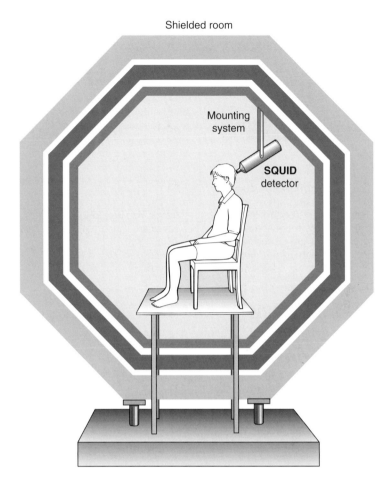

Shielded room

Mounting
system

SQUID
detector

Fig. 2.4 Shielded room used for studying the magnetic field of the
brain. The SQUID detector is positioned close to but not touching the
subject's head. Clothing must be free of magnetic material, such as
zippers or nails in shoes. Shielded rooms such as this were
manufactured by Takenaka Corporation. Illustration redrawn from
Takenaka website: http://www.takenaka.co.jp/takenaka_e/techno/
19_sldrm/19_sldrm.htm and used by kind permission of Nodoru
Uenishi, Takenaka Corporation, New York

Because the first measurements were technically difficult to accomplish, the
focus was on the alpha rhythm, which is a strong component of the brain
waves. It is much easier to demonstrate strong alpha rhythms when the eyes
are closed (Fig. 2.5A). (In later chapters we will return to the possible role of
the alpha rhythm in healing.)

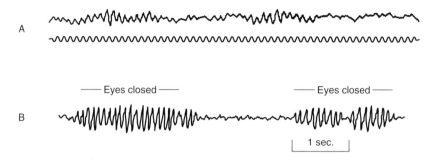

Eyes closed ——   —— Eyes closed ——

1 sec.

Fig. 2.5 Electroencephalograms. **A.** The first published electroencephalogram of a human being. The lower line is a time pulse at 10 cycles per second. (After Berger 1929.) **B.** The alpha rhythm of the human electroencephalogram. The waves are much easier to observe when the eyes are closed. (After Adrian et al 1934.) Cohen (1972) found that the magnetoencephalograms recorded with a SQUID magnetometer are similar to electrical recordings such as these.

Weak vs strong fields

When Einthoven discovered the electric field of the heart, it was an extremely weak field and very difficult to measure. Because of progress in instrumentation, we now recognize that the heart produces the strongest field in the body. In comparison to the heart fields, the fields of the brain are weak. However, neural activities control our movements and attitudes about ourselves, and can therefore produce profound effects. Hence 'strong vs weak' is more a statement about measuring instruments than about the biological importance of the different fields.

Measurement of the biomagnetic fields of the heart and brain led to a veritable explosion of research into biomagnetics. It turned out that biomagnetic fields are often more indicative of events taking place within the body than are electrical measurements at the skin surface. For example, biomagnetic fields produced by the brain pass undistorted through the cerebrospinal fluid (CSF), across the connective tissue covering of the brain (the dura), and through the skull bones and scalp. These tissues are virtually transparent to magnetic fields. In contrast, the electrical signals recorded with the electroencephalogram become distorted, smeared, and decreased in strength by a factor of about 10 000 as they pass through the surrounding tissues. EEGs therefore do not give as precise a representation of brain activity as MEGs. Electrical measurements are also compromised by complex interactions between the skin and the electrode pickups, which can act as batteries and generate currents on their own. All in all, the MEG appears to provide more detail and better spatial localization than the EEG.

Scientists realized that all of the classical electrical diagnostic tools have biomagnetic equivalents. For example, the eye acts as a battery and produces a substantial electrical field whose intensity depends on the amount of light falling on the retina. Records of this field are called electroretinograms. The magnetoretinogram is the corresponding record of the retina's biomagnetic field in the space around the head.

Contractions of other muscles besides the heart produce electrical fields that are recorded by electromyography. The corresponding magnetic recordings are called magnetomyograms. Every muscle in the body produces magnetic pulses when it contracts. The larger muscles produce larger fields and the smaller muscles, such as those that move and focus the eye, produce very tiny fields. This fact may be of interest to movement therapists, because we now know that any movement of any part of the body is 'broadcast' into the space around the body as a precise 'biomagnetic signature' of that movement. The relative strengths of the various biomagnetic fields produced by the human body are shown in Figure 2.6.

SQUID instruments are now available commercially from more than a dozen manufacturers, and are being used in medical research laboratories all over the world to explore aspects of the biological fields that scientists were certain did not exist a few decades ago (for a review, see Hämäläinen et al 1993). Some of

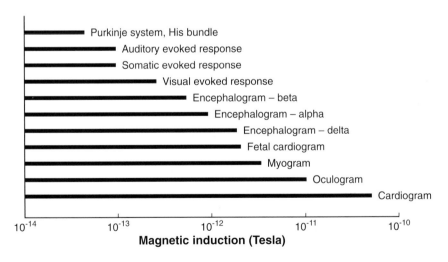

Fig. 2.6 The relative strength of the various biomagnetic fields measured in the spaces around the human body. (Based on data presented in Fig. 1 of Williamson & Kaufman 1981.)

the exciting work involves using arrays of SQUID detectors that can produce three-dimensional maps of the fields around the body.

Effects of practice on brain waves

An example of a recent study is an investigation of the magnetic brain waves of musicians such as violinists and other string players (Elbert et al 1995). Practicing and performing with these instruments involves considerable manual dexterity and sensory processing, particularly in fingering with the left hand. In comparison, the thumb of the left hand grasps the neck of the instrument. While the position and pressure of the thumb are frequently shifted, far less dexterity is required. And the tasks of the right hand, which manipulates the bow, also involve fewer precise finger movements. The hypothesis was that repeated and intense use of the fingers of the left hand, over years of practice, would increase the size of brain areas involved in movements and sensation of those fingers. Six violinists, two cellists, and a guitarist were studied. Six non-musicians served as controls.

Using an array of SQUID detectors such as the one shown in Figure 2.7, the investigators were able to map the surface or cortex of the brain, and show that the biomagnetic fields produced by specific cortical regions were more intense in string musicians compared to non-performers. There was also a correlation between the number of years of practice and the intensity of the brain waves from the areas controlling skilled fingers. The number of nerve cells involved in controlling and sensing movement seems to increase with practice. This is just one of many studies completed or in progress that are enabling scientists to map the biomagnetic fields of the human body on a moment-to-moment basis, and to determine how biofields correlate with physiological processes.

Hypothesis

It would obviously be fascinating to know if repeatedly practicing 'hands-on' methods – massage, Rolfing® or structural integration, Trager, reflexology, acupuncture, shiatsu, QiGong, etc. – enhances the biomagnetic output from corresponding areas of the brain, as practicing with a musical instrument does. This is a hypothesis worthy of testing.

The brain field, like the heart field, is not confined to the organ that produces it. We refer to 'brain waves' as though they are confined to the brain, but they are not. The fields of all of the organs spread throughout the body and into

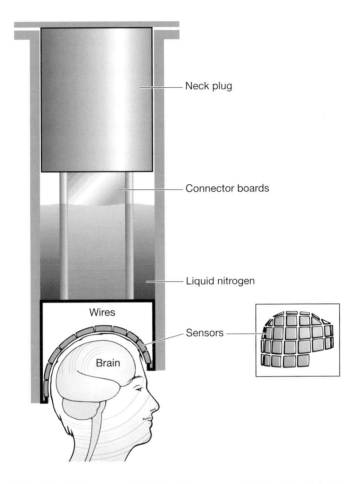

Fig. 2.7 The 122-channel SQUID, 'Neuromag-122' built in Helsinki. The sensors are wrapped around the head as shown. A similar device was used by Elbert and colleagues in 1995 to measure the brain magnetic fields of string musicians. Practice in fingering the instruments is correlated with a strong brain field, particularly for those cortical regions associated with using and sensing with the fingers of the left hand. (After Hämäläinen et al 1993, Fig. 41, p. 467, with permission from Reviews of Modern Physics and Dr Risto Ilmoniemi.)

the space around it. One of the primary channels for the flow of electrical waves through the body is the circulatory system. So one could hypothesize that practicing 'hands-on' work can also affect the biomagnetic output from a therapist's fingers and hands. In other words, *all* forms of therapeutic contact may involve far more than simple pressure on the skin.

Biomagnetic fields and senses

From the research done over the last few decades, we can definitely conclude that:

◆ Living organisms have biomagnetic fields around them.

◆ These fields change from moment to moment in relation to events taking place inside the body.

◆ These fields give a clearer representation of what is going on in the body than classical electrical diagnostic tools such as the electrocardiogram and the electro-encephalogram.

This should not be taken to suggest that the 'fields of life' are entirely magnetic. Other kinds of fields are also present (see Ch. 6).

It is one thing to say the biofields accurately represent events taking place inside the body, and another for a person to claim they can see or feel those fields. However, it has now been predicted and shown that Josephson effects, the basis for the SQUID magnetic detector, also exist in living tissues (Del Giudice et al 1989).

There is an old idea that our technology recapitulates our biology – that all of our technological devices were first invented and perfected during millions of years of evolutionary experimentation with the laws and energies of nature. Perhaps there is a magnetic sense in the human body, a sense that can be developed and used in healing.

We shall explore the application of biomagnetism in polarity therapy and related methods in subsequent chapters. First, though, we need to examine the circuits through which energy moves in the body, and the kinds of energy that are involved.

References

Adrian ED, Matthews BHC 1934 The Berger rhythm: potential changes from the occipital lobes in man. Brain 57(4):24–385

Anderson P W, Rowell J M 1963 Probable observation of the Josephson superconducting tunneling effect. Physical Review Letters 10:230–232

Baule G M, McFee R 1963 Detection of the magnetic field of the heart. American Heart Journal 66:95–96

Berger H 1929 Uber das Elektrenkephalogramm des Menschen. Archiv fur Psykchiatrica 87:527–570

Brockmeier K, Burghoff M, Koch H, Schmitz L, Zimmerman R 1995.

ST segment changes in a healthy subject during pharmacological stress test using magnetocardiographic and electrocardiographic multichannel recordings. In: Baumgartner C, Deecke L, Stroink G, Williamson S J (eds) Biomagnetism: fundamental research and clinical applications. Proceedings of the 9th International Conference on Biomagnetism. Studies in Applied Electromagnetics and Mechanics Vol 7. Elsevier Science, IOS Press, Amsterdam, pp 633–636

Cohen D 1967 Magnetic fields around the torso: production by electrical activity of the human heart. Science 156:652–654

Cohen D 1972 Magnetoencephalography: detection of the brain's electrical activity with a superconducting magnetometer. Science 175:664–666

Cohen D, Edelsack E A, Zimmerman J E 1970 Magnetocardiograms taken inside a shielded room with a superconducting point-contact magnetometer. Applied Physics Letters 16:278–280

Day W 1989 Bridge from nowhere: a story of space, motion, and the structure of matter. House of Talos, East Lansing, Michigan

Day W 1996 Bridge from nowhere II. Rhombics Press, Cambridge, MA

Del Giudice E S, Doglia S, Milani M, Smith J M, Vitiello G 1989 Magnetic flux quantization and Josephson behaviour in living systems. Physica Scripta 40:786–791

Einthoven W 1906 Le télécardiogramme. Archives Internationales de Physiologie 4:132–164

Elbert T, Pantev C, Weinbruch C, Rockstroh B, Taub E 1995 Increased cortical representation of the fingers of the left hand in string players. Science 270:305–307

Hämäläinen M, Hari R, Ilmoniemi R J, Knuutila J, Lounasmaa O V 1993 Magnetoencephalography: theory, instrumentation, and applications to noninvasive studies of the working human brain. Reviews of Modern Physics 65:413–497

Kaufman L, Okada Y, Tripp J, Weinberg H 1984 Evoked neuromagnetic fields. Annals of the New York Academy of Sciences 425:728

Josephson B D 1962 Possible new effects in superconductive tunneling. Physics Letters 1:251–253

Josephson B D 1965 Supercurrents through barriers. Advances in Physics 14:419–451

Langenberg D N, Scalapino D J, Taylor B N 1966 The Josephson effects. Scientific American 214:30–39

Shapiro S 1963 Josephson currents in superconducting tunneling: the effect of microwaves and other observations. Physical Review Letters 11:80–82

Williamson S J Kaufman L 1981 Biomagnetism. Journal of Magnetism and Magnetic Materials 22:129–201, p. 132

Wolff M 1993 Fundamental laws, microphysics, and cosmology. Physics Essays 6:181–203

Wolff M 1997 Exploring the universe and the origin of its laws. Frontier Perspectives 6(2):44–56

Zimmerman J E 1972 Josephson effect devices and low frequency field sensing. Cryogenics 12:19–31

Zimmerman J E, Thiene P, Harding J T 1970 Design and operation of stable rf-biased superconducting point-contact quantum devices, and a note on the properties of perfectly clean metal contacts. Journal of Applied Physics 41:1572–1580

3 The 'circuitry' of the body

Nature has neither kernel nor shell – she is everything at once.
Goethe

When we look at any one thing in the world, we find it is hitched to everything else.
John Muir

The moment one gives close attention to anything, even a blade of grass, it becomes a mysterious, awesome, indescribably magnificent world in itself.
Henry Miller

The historical background presented in Chapter 1 explains why the various energetic therapies have received little attention from Western biomedicine. The main intellectual issue is the long-standing contention over 'vitalism vs mechanism'. Chapter 2 described how biomagnetic fields have been detected in the spaces around the body. Mention was made of the laws of physics that state that when charges flow, magnetic fields are created in the surrounding spaces.

Now we need to explore precisely where the charges are flowing, and how those flows are influenced by diseases and disorders. We shall see that there are, indeed, energetic circuits in the living organism. Energy and information stream through these circuits to every nook and cranny of the body. These flows can be influenced by subtle energies in the environment. Moreover, disease and disorder alter these flows in predictable ways.

The fundamental discoveries providing the basis for the various energetic therapies have taken place in a wide variety of disciplines. With a few exceptions, the remarkable generalizations – the 'big picture' – emerging from the individual discoveries has been virtually invisible to the participants in the search for knowledge. What has been discovered is the scientific basis for the interconnectedness and continuity of the parts of the living organism. This interconnectedness is based upon careful study of the structure and function of cells and tissues. It provides a basis for the streaming of energy and information throughout the living body.

Electricity vs electronics

Before beginning our exploration, it is important to clarify the distinction between biological electricity and biological electronics.

Biological electricity is a large-scale phenomenon arising from the movements of charged ions such as sodium, potassium, chloride, calcium, and magnesium. In virtually all cases, the electricity arises because of the large electrical polarity across cell membranes, and the ability of these membranes to temporarily depolarize and then repolarize. This is the process that enables nerves to conduct signals from place to place within the body. A wave of depolarization also goes along a muscle cell, and triggers it to contract. The large fields and measurable magnetic fields picked up from the heart, retina, muscles, and brain arise primarily because of the electrical currents that flow as they carry out their activities. Less known but just as important are slow waves of electrical depolarization that are set up across the skin in response to injury. These are called injury potentials, and they are important in triggering tissue repair.

Biological electricity is widely studied by many different kinds of scientists, including electrobiologists, physiologists, and neurophysiologists. Much is known about the subject because electrical currents are relatively easy to measure.

In contrast, biological electronics is a relatively new subject of research. It deals with the flows of much smaller entities than ions. These are mainly electrons, protons, and the spaces where an electron is missing, called a *hole*.

For a familiar example, consider the electrical appliances in your home, and the wiring that brings electrical power to them. Contrast this with the far more subtle electronic processes taking place within your computer or television. These devices contain electronic circuits that utilize far smaller amounts of power to carry out sophisticated tasks at very high speed. This is possible because of advances in solid state physics and electronics and the use of semiconductor devices. We are now going to look at the corresponding subtle circuitry that has been discovered in living systems. We begin by taking a close look at cells.

Cell structure and the 'living matrix'

One of the most important developments in recent science is a better under-standing of the structure and energetics of the material substrate of the body – the living substance that is touched and interacted with in all therapeutic approaches. For the hands-on therapist, the energetic properties of this living substance have both conceptual and practical consequences. To understand the new developments, we begin with breakthroughs in our understandings of the cell.

A few decades ago, the living cell was visualized as a membrane-bound bag containing a solution of molecules. Figure 3.1A shows a cell as it is often illustrated in texts. Note that the cell is embedded in a fibrous material, called the connective tissue or extracellular matrix. This matrix contains large amounts of a fascinating protein called collagen. Most of the cell interior appears 'empty' in the drawing. Illustrations like this are still widely used today, even though they omit one of the most important attributes of cell structure.

The main reason the image shown in Figure 3.1A has persisted, and can still be found in modern texts, is that most biochemists were in agreement that life consists of a sequence of chemical reactions taking place in a 'soup' or solution within the cell. For example, consider glycolysis, the sequential breakdown of sugar molecules by 10 'soluble' enzymes (Fig. 3.1B): Glycolysis and other bio-chemical pathways were discovered with techniques in which tissues and cells were broken apart. Centrifugation was then used to separate the dissolved mole-cules from the solids, which were discarded because they were not considered important.

The biochemical image of life is as follows: there are 'particles', the enzymes, proteins, amino acids, sugars, etc., that randomly diffuse about within the enclosed volume of the cell. When appropriate molecules chance to bump into each other, they interact, and chemical bonds are formed or broken. In this way, chemical energy is liberated, living structures are assembled or taken apart, toxins are broken down, and life's activities are carried out. Figure 3.1C represents this 'random walk' image of the steps in glycolysis.

Early electron microscopy confirmed that cells contain substantial amounts of 'empty' space. It was assumed that this is where the particles are dissolved or suspended, and where metabolism takes place.

The torrent of information and clinical applications developed from this 'molecular soup' view of the cell led to an attitude that 'there are only a few

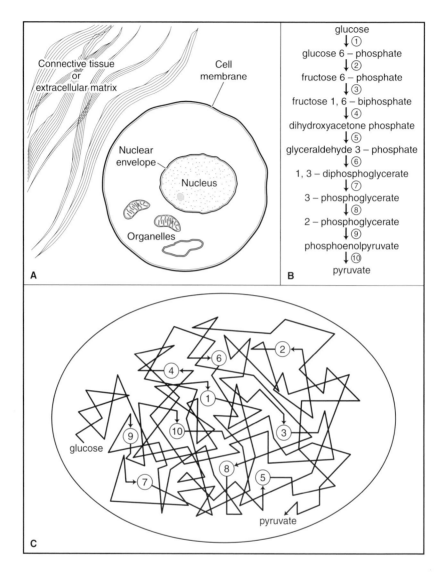

Fig. 3.1 The cell and 'solution biochemistry.' **A** A cell as it is often illustrated in texts. Most of the cell interior appears 'empty.' Illustrations like this are still widely used today, even though they omit some of the most important attributes of cell structure. Note that the cell is embedded in a fibrous material, called the connective tissue or extracellular matrix. This matrix contains large amounts of a fascinating protein called collagen. **B** An enzymatic pathway, glycolysis, as it is usually depicted in texts. The 10 glycolytic enzymes convert glucose into pyruvate in a series of steps. **C** The 'bag of solution' model of the cell. The 10 enzymes of glycolysis float about in the solution, and reactants randomly diffuse about until they chance to bump into the next enzyme in the sequence. The probability of locating the next enzyme is enhanced because there are many copies of each enzyme floating about. However, the delays built into the system make it a relatively slow process.

problems remaining, and we will soon be able to answer all of them, using this same, incredibly successful, approach'. Physiologists seized the 'bag of solution' model of cell structure, and conducted decades of research in which an underlying assumption was that substances crossing a layer of cells, such as the intestinal wall, simply diffuse through the fluid compartments inside the cells.

The cell is not a bag

This picture is changing slowly but dramatically because of the discovery that the cell is *not* a bag of solution. The more closely biologists and microscopists looked at cells, the more structures they found. With better preparation techniques, electron microscopists began to see within cells the material that the biochemists had been discarding when they purified the 'soluble' enzymes.

We now know that the cell is so filled with filaments and tubes and fibres and trabeculae – collectively called the cytoplasmic matrix or cytoskeleton – that there is little space left for a solution of randomly diffusing 'billiard ball' molecules (Fig. 3.2). Moreover, there is very little water inside cells that can dissolve the so-called soluble enzymes. Virtually all the cell water is bound in particular ways to the cellular framework (see e.g. Cope 1967, Corongiu & Clementi 1981, Ling 1992, Damadian 1971).

Many of the enzymes that were previously thought to be floating about within the cytoplasmic 'soup' are actually attached to structures within the cell and nucleus (see inset to Fig. 3.2, Oschman 1984, Ingber 1993). These attachments are delicate. Biochemical homogenization techniques detach enzymes and other proteins from the cellular and nuclear scaffolds that support them in actual living cells. 'Solution biochemistry', while quite instructive, is an artifact: 'the empirical fact that a given molecule appears primarily in the "soluble" fraction may divert attention from the cataclysmic violence of the most gentle homogenization procedure' (McConkey 1982).

Most textbooks still oversimplify biochemistry by showing metabolic pathways as linear sequences of steps (Fig. 3.1B), without mentioning the essential *structural* or *solid state* context in which the chemistry of life takes place.

Continuum

Soon after the cytoskeleton became a popular subject for research, it was realized that the cellular matrix is connected, across the cell surface, with the connective tissue system or extracellular matrix (also shown in Fig. 3.2). A whole class of

A

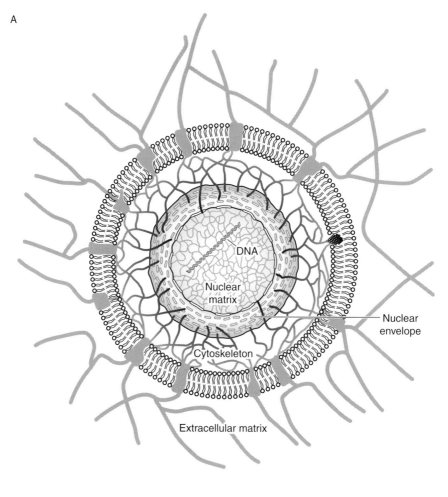

B Glucose

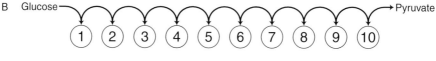

Pyruvate

Fig. 3.2 **A** Contemporary image of a cell and its relations: the living matrix. Modern cell biology has recognized that the cell interior is virtually filled with fibers and tubes and filaments, collectively called the cytoskeleton or cytoplasmic matrix. Likewise, the nucleus contains a nuclear matrix that supports the genetic material. Linkers called integrins extend across the cell surface, connecting the cytoskeleton with the extracellular matrix. The entire system is termed the living matrix. **B** Shows a more realistic model of a biochemical pathway, glycolysis, in which the enzymes are organized in sequence along the cytoskeletal structure. The reaction sequence can proceed very rapidly because reactants are passed from one enzyme to the next to the next, as in an assembly line.

'trans-membrane' linking molecules, or 'integrins,' has been discovered. Likewise, it is now recognized that the cytoplasmic matrix also links to the nuclear envelope, nuclear matrix, and genes.

Conceptually, these discoveries are profoundly important. The boundaries between the cell environment, the cell interior, and the genetic material are not as sharp or as impermeable as we once thought. As a hands-on therapist, what you touch is not merely the skin – you contact a continuous interconnected webwork that extends throughout the body. Indeed, the skin is one of the first tissues in which this continuity was documented (Fig. 3.3, Ellison & Garrod, 1984).

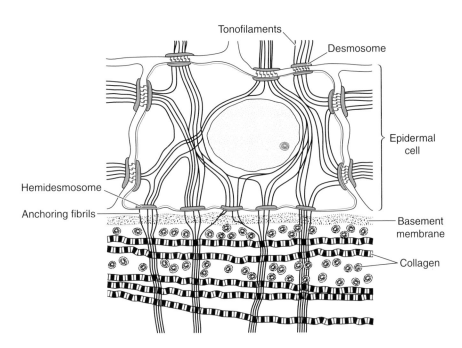

Fig. 3.3 The epidermal–dermal continuum. Ellison and Garrod (1984) and others cited by them have described the epidermal–dermal junction in detail. Adjacent epidermal cells are attached to each other by desmosomes, and are anchored to the dermal connective tissue by hemidesmosomes. All of the anchors are traversed by tonofilaments, which form a continuous fibrous matrix joining together all epidermal cells throughout the skin. Anchoring fibrils link the cellular matrix with the connective tissue. The dermal connective tissue is part of a continuous integrated system extending throughout the body. The cytoskeletons of all other cells in the body are similarly linked to the connective tissue system. (After Ellison & Garrod 1984, Fig. 10, p.170, with kind permission from the Journal of Cell Science and the Company of Biologists, Ltd.)

The entire interconnected system has been called the connective tissue/cytoskeleton (Oschman 1994), the tissue-tensegrity matrix (see Ch. 4) (Pienta & Coffey 1991), or, simply, *the living matrix*. A popular acupuncture text refers to 'the web that has no weaver' (Kaptchuk 1983).

The living matrix is a continuous and dynamic 'supramolecular' webwork, extending into every nook and cranny of the body: a nuclear matrix within a cellular matrix within a connective tissue matrix. In essence, when you touch a human body, you are touching a continuously interconnected system, composed of virtually all of the molecules in the body linked together in an intricate webwork. The living matrix has no fundamental unit or central aspect, no part that is primary or most basic. The properties of the whole net depend upon the integrated activities of all of the components. Effects on one part of the system can, and do spread to others.

This is an important image of the structure of the living body. Our images shape our therapeutic successes because they can give rise to specific intentions. Intentions are not trivial, because they give rise to specific patterns of electrical and magnetic activity in the nervous system of the therapist that can spread through their body and into the body of a patient. We shall return to this subject later (Chs 8 and 15).

While it is obviously useful to study the various parts and systems of the body, each component can be regarded as a local domain or subdivision of a continuous web. The shape, form, mechanical, energetic, and functional characteristics of every cell, tissue, or organ arise because of local variations in the properties of the matrix. The genome, within the nuclear matrix, is a subdivision of this network.

Information flows

A legacy of the mechanism/vitalism argument and the reductionistic approach was a tendency to disregard the overall coordination or integration of the body, such as the systemic regulations proposed in acupuncture theory. By its very nature, the reductionist approach assumes that it is virtually impossible to study phenomena at the level of the whole organism, simply because it is too complex. To make sense out of it, life must be taken apart and studied one piece at a time. The reassembly of the parts into a whole is a process that must be put off until some vague and distant future date, when we have come to understand all of the parts. A 'general systems theory' was developed (von Bertalanffy 1971), but few physiologists took an interest in it.

Nonetheless, in order to survive, complex living systems require an intricate web of informational processes. Each component must be able to quickly and appropriately adjust its activities in relation to what the other parts are doing. One distinguished physiologist, Edward F. Adolph, took a deep look at the mechanisms of physiological integration: 'The biology of wholeness is the study of the body as an integrated, coordinated, successful system. No parts or properties are uncorrelated, all are demonstrably interlinked. And the links are not single chains, but a great number of crisscrossed pathways' (Adolph 1982).

When scientists think of regulations, they usually begin with the nervous system. The discovery of neurohormones led to an understanding of how neural and hormonal systems interact. Chemical regulations are usually viewed in the same manner as cell metabolism – i.e. controlling substances (hormones) diffuse through the extracellular matrix, until they happen to bump into 'target' cells, upon which they exert their influences.

A simplistic view is that some hormones react with cell surfaces, while others cross the cell membrane and exert their effects on the cell interior. We now know that many hormones deliver messages to cell surfaces, and that this then causes the production of 'second messengers' within the cells that activate cellular activities (see e.g. Rasmussen 1981). Hence, communications in living systems involve two main languages: chemical and energetic. Chemical regulations are carried out by hormones, various 'factors' (e.g. growth factor, epithelial growth factor, etc.) and the various 'second messengers' within cells. As stated above, energetic interactions are of two kinds, electrical and electronic. The electrical activities of nerves and muscles are well known, but there are many other kinds of energetic signaling systems. Some remain to be discovered.

We shall see that an even more profound realization is emerging. The entire living matrix is simultaneously a mechanical, vibrational or oscillatory, energetic, electronic, and informational network (Pienta & Coffey 1991, Oschman 1994). Hence the entire composite of physiological and regulatory processes we refer to as 'the living state' take place within the context of a continuous living matrix.

A sensible design for a living system is one in which every cell receives information on the activities taking place in every other part of the body:

> The integrated human body is the sum of thousands of physiological
> processes and traits working together. Each breath and each heartbeat
> involves the working together of countless events. Huge numbers of

functions are carried on simultaneously. The parts and processes within an organism are woven together with great intricacy. Coordination occurs at a thousand points. If there were no integration of activities, life would be a random jumble of physical and chemical events that reaches no known accomplishment. In actuality, each process is of consequence to the whole. (Adolph 1982)

Physiological integration is possible because every cell and every molecule fine-tunes its activities appropriately. While the diffusion of chemicals from place to place is one important means of communication, it is too slow a process to account for the rapid and subtle aspects of the living process. We are now discerning that the living matrix itself is a high-speed communication network linking every part with every other.

Matrix dynamics: signaling and cell crawling

Recently there has been tremendous excitement in the research community about the properties of the living matrix. The excitement arises because the matrix has key roles in defense and repair. Moreover, it is through this matrix that nutrients, hormones and other signal molecules, toxins, and waste products diffuse to and from all cells. Obviously the properties of this system, its 'openness' to the flows of various materials, is essential to life.

One of the conclusions from studying the various complementary therapies in relation to conventional medicine is that the latter has become focused on the various organs and systems and given relatively scant attention to the ways in which they communicate with each other via the living matrix. In contrast, complementary therapists often solve health problems by first attending to the 'quality' of the matrix, meaning the way the flesh looks and feels to the touch.

The molecules that link the cell interior with the extracellular matrix have come to be called *integrins*: 'Integrins are a class of adhesion molecules that "glue" cells in place. Surprisingly, at a fundamental level, they also regulate most functions of the body. The author reveals the hidden role of integrins in arthritis, heart disease, stroke, osteoporosis and the spread of cancer' (introduction to Horwitz 1997).

The living matrix is a dynamic rather than a fixed system. The connections between adjacent cells, and between the cells and the substrate, are labile rather than permanent. Connections form, break, and reform as cells change shape and/or crawl about. Specific connectors, called tonofilaments, desmosomes, hemidesmosomes, integrins, connexins, and anchoring filaments, are all labile structures that can disconnect, retract, dissolve, and reform (Gabbiani et al 1978, Krawczyk & Wilgram 1973). These reversible adhesions enable epidermal cells, fibroblasts, osteoblasts, myoblasts, and other 'generative' cells to move about when necessary to repair (re-epithialize) damaged skin and restore other tissues. Ameboid motions enable leukocytes to migrate to sites of infection, or into tumors for resorption of 'non-self' material.

Solid state biochemistry

As discussed above, biochemistry was founded on the study of reactions taking place in solution. The discovery of the cytoskeleton, with its dynamic inter-connections with the nuclear and connective tissue matrices, has advanced our understanding of *solid state biochemistry*.

The development of this field obviously does not reject the beautiful and profoundly important work done by biochemists and molecular biologists on the 'soluble' enzymes and their activities. Instead, solid state biochemistry opens up the study of additional processes taking place on and in the solid fibers and filaments that constitute living cells and tissues. This approach also opens up a deeper understanding of the effects of hands-on, structural, energetic, and biomechanical therapies on processes taking place throughout the body.

Solution biochemistry required that the molecules within the cell diffuse about more or less randomly until they bump into appropriate enzymes (Fig. 3.1C). Solid state biochemistry recognizes that chemical reactions proceed in a much more orderly and rapid manner if they are organized on a structural frame-work (inset of Fig. 3.2). Moreover, the living matrix concept opens up the possibilities for global control: signals traveling *in* the matrix can regulate or fine-tune matrix-associated enzymes throughout the organism. Here we distin-guish between messages that travel *through* the matrix, as by diffusion through the interstitial fluid lying between its fibers, and messages traveling *in* the matrix itself, as by electronic conduction along the protein backbone, or by hopping of protons in the layers of water associated with the protein surface (Ho & Knight 1998). The mechanisms involved in matrix communication are dealt with in the next sections.

To understand the therapeutic significance of solid state biochemistry and matrix regulation, we begin with an examination of the high degree of order, or regularity, or crystallinity present in cells and tissues.

Crystalline arrays in cells and tissues: piezoelectricity

> Form, in contradistinction to random shape, contains parts or elements in a definite, characteristically recurrent array in space. Thus form is the result of the orderly manner in which those elements are combined and arranged. Form of a higher order of complexity accordingly can emerge from the ordered assembly of simpler formed elements of mutual fit. (Weiss 1965)

We do not intuitively consider biological materials to be crystalline, because when we think of crystals we usually think of hard materials, like diamond or agate. Living crystals are composed of long, thin, pliable molecules, and are soft and flexible. To be more precise, they are liquid crystals (e.g. Bouligand 1978).

Crystalline arrangements are the rule and not the exception in living systems. Figure 3.4 gives some important examples. Physicists know a great deal about the properties of crystals. The information they have obtained is of considerable medical importance. For example, certain kinds of crystals are piezoelectric, that is they generate electric fields when they are compressed or stretched.

Physiologists are aware of this, and have studied the generation of electricity by bone. Each step you take compresses bones in the legs and elsewhere, and generates characteristic electrical fields. The piezoelectric effect is not, however, confined to bone. Virtually all of the tissues in the body generate electric fields when they are compressed or stretched (Oschman 1981). The piezoelectric effect is partly responsible for these electric fields. Another source of such fields is a phenomenon known as streaming potentials. The relative contribution of these two ways of generating electric fields in tissues is under investigation (e.g. MacGinitie 1995). Figure 3.5 compares the two phenomena.

The important point is that when a bone or cartilage is compressed, when a tendon or ligament stretches, or when the skin is stretched or bent, as at a joint, minute electric pulsations are set up. These oscillations, and their harmonics, are precisely representative of the forces acting on the tissues involved. In other words, they contain information on the precise nature of the movements taking place. This information is electrically and electronically conducted through the surrounding living matrix. One of the roles of this information is in the control of form.

The control of body structure

The therapeutic and physiological importance of the piezoelectric and other electronic properties of tissues is that they provide a framework for under-

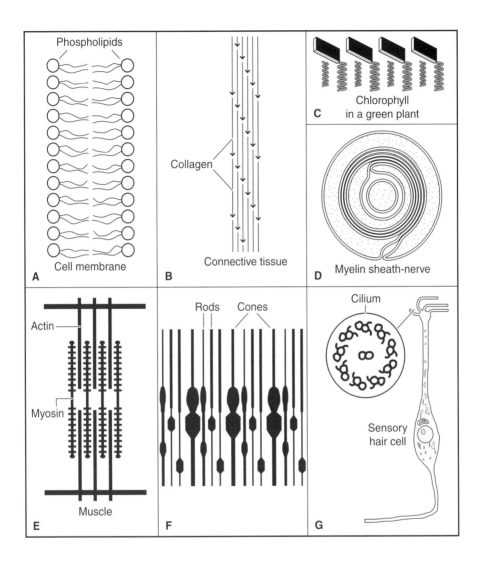

Fig. 3.4 Crystalline arrangements in various tissues. Crystalline arrangements are the rule and not the exception in living systems. **A** Arrays of phospholipid molecules form cell membranes. **B** Collagen arrays form connective tissue. **C** Arrays of chlorophyll molecules in the leaf. **D** The myelin sheath of nerves. Each layer is composed of membranes such as shown in A. (After Fawcett 1994, Fig. 11.21, p.335, with permission from Chapman & Hall.) **E** The contractile array in muscle, composed of actin and myosin molecules organized around each other. **F** The array of sensory endings in the retina. **G** arrays of microtubules, microfilaments, and other fibrous components of the cytoskeleton occur in nerves and other kinds of cells. Here are the cilia of sensory organs such as those responsible for detecting odors and sound.

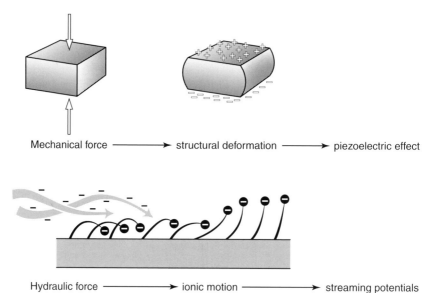

Mechanical force ⟶ structural deformation ⟶ piezoelectric effect

Hydraulic force ⟶ ionic motion ⟶ streaming potentials

Fig. 3.5 Two methods by which movements generate electricity in tissues. The upper drawing shows the generation of piezoelectric or pressure electricity by the deformation of a crystalline structure. The lower drawing shows the way streaming potentials are developed by the flow of fluid containing charged ions over electrically charged surfaces. The charge is built up by the electrostatic interactions between the fixed tissue charge and the mobile charge. Potentials of this type are generated by both blood flow and propulsion of extracellular fluids through the extracellular matrix, as a result of tissue deformation. The streaming potentials can interact additively or subtractively with piezoelectric potentials. (After Bassett 1978, with permission from Harcourt Publishers.)

standing how the body adapts to the ways it is used (Oschman 1989). It has long been recognized that bones and other elements of connective tissue are constantly remodeling in response to the loads imposed upon them. From the biochemical perspective, this is referred to as 'metabolic regeneration', a process discovered and documented by Schoenheimer and colleagues over half a century ago (Schoenheimer 1942, Ratner 1979).

The electric fields produced during movements are widely considered to provide the information that directs the activities of 'generative' cells (e.g. Bassett 1971, Bassett et al 1964). These are the osteoblasts, myoblasts, perivascular cells, fibroblasts, and other 'stem' cells that lay down or resorb collagen and thereby reform tissues so they can adapt to the ways the body is used. This regulatory concept dates to Wolff in 1892 (see Bassett 1968):

Wolff's law

'The form of the bone (or other connective tissue) being given, the bone elements (collagen) place or displace themselves in the direction of the functional pressure and increase or decrease their mass to reflect the amount of functional pressure'.

Again, these concepts are highly relevant to the hands-on, energetic, or movement therapist. They provide the basis for progressive changes in body structure that take place because of the ways in which individuals use their bodies in relation to gravity, because of habits or injuries. They also provide a basis for the restorative measures that can be used to correct gravity-related disorders (Rolf 1962, Oschman 1997) (see Ch. 11).

Properties of the living matrix

On the basis of the information presented so far, we can begin to form a picture of the energetic systems in the living body. The living matrix continuum includes all of the connective tissues and cytoskeletons of all of the cells, throughout the body. We can summarize its properties as follows:

◆ All of the great systems of the body – the circulation, the nervous system, the musculoskeletal system, the digestive tract, the various organs and glands – are everywhere covered with material that is but a part of a continuous connective tissue fabric.

◆ The connective tissues form a mechanical continuum, extending throughout the animal body, even into the innermost parts of each cell.

◆ The connective tissues determine the overall shape of the organism as well as the detailed architecture of its parts.

◆ All movement, of the body as a whole or of its smallest parts, is created by tensions carried through the connective tissue fabric.

◆ Each tension, each compression, each movement causes the crystalline lattice of the connective tissues to generate bioelectronic signals that are precisely characteristic of those tensions, compressions, and movements.

◆ The connective tissue fabric is a semiconducting communication network that can carry the bioelectronic signals between every part of the body and every other part.

Circuits and meridians

That the human body comprises electronic circuits is not widely appreciated, and this is part of the reason some of the phenomena found in alternative medicine have been difficult to grasp. Electronic circuits can be designed to do many things – this is the wonder of our present age of technology. It is seldom understood that life has tested all possible combinations of quantum electronic tricks and has mastered all of them for its purposes, through the

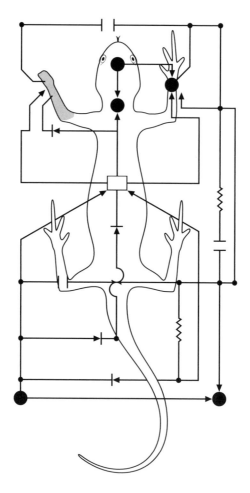

Fig. 3.6 Logo for a conference entitled 'Mechanisms of Growth Control, Clinical Applications', held on September 26–28, 1979, at the State University of New York Upstate Medical Center.
An electronic circuit is superimposed over the body of a salamander, a popular animal for research on regeneration.

honing process of evolution. The next chapter will take up the discovery of the electronic properties of living matter.

Information about biological electronics has been with us for a long time, but it has not been widely appreciated. Figure 3.6 shows the image of a circuit diagram laid over a salamander which was used as the logo for a scientific conference on mechanisms of growth control, clinical applications, held at the State University of New York Upstate Medical Center in 1979.

The best introduction to the electronic circuitry of the human body is to be found in the study of acupuncture. We take a close look at this in Chapter 5, after the next chapter, which looks at some discoveries that help explain how energy and information circulate within the 'living matrix'.

References

Adolph EF, 1982 Physiological Integrations in Action. Physiologist 25(2) (April) Supplement

Bassett CAL 1968 Biologic significance of piezoelectricity. Calcified Tissue Research 1:252–272

Bassett CAL 1971 Effect of forces on skeletal tissues. In: Downey JA, Darling RC (eds) Physiological basis of rehabilitation medicine. W.B. Saunders, Philadelphia, pp. 283–316

Bassett CAL 1978 Pulsing electromagnetic fields: a new approach to surgical problems. In: Buchwald H, Varco RL (eds) Metabolic surgery. Grune & Stratton, New York, ch. 11, p 260

Bassett CAL, Pawluk, RJ, Becker RO 1964 Effects of electric currents on bone formation in vivo. Nature (London):204:652–654

von Bertalanffy L 1971 General system theory. Foundations, development, applications (revised and enlarged edition). Penguin, London

Bouligand Y 1978 Liquid crystals and their analogs in biological systems. In: Liebert L (ed) Liquid crystals. Solid State Physics 14 (supplement):259–294

Cope FW 1967 A theory of cell hydration governed by adsorption of water on cell proteins rather than by osmotic pressure. Bulletin of Mathematical Biophysics 29:583–596

Corongiu G, Clementi E 1981 Simulations of the solvent structure for macromolecules. I. Solvation of B-DNA double helix at T=300 K. Biopolymers 20:551–571

Damadian R 1971 Tumor detection by nuclear magnetic resonance. Science 171(19):1151–1153

Ellison J, Garrod DR 1984 Anchoring filaments of the amphibian epidermal junction traverse the basal lamina entirely from the plasma membrane of hemidesmosomes to the dermis. Journal of Cell Science 72:163–172

Fawcett DW 1994 A textbook of histology, 12th edn. Chapman & Hall, New York

Gabbiani G, Chaponnier C, Huttner I 1978 Cytoplasmic filaments and gap junctions in epithelial cells and myofibroblasts during wound healing. Journal of Cell Biology 76(3):561–568

Ho M-W, Knight DP 1998 The acupuncture system and the liquid crystalline collagen fibers of the connective tissues. American Journal of Chinese Medicine 26(3–4):1–13

Horwitz AF 1997 Integrins and health. Discovered only recently, these adhesive cell surface molecules have quickly revealed themselves to be critical to proper functioning of the body and to life itself. Scientific American 276:68–75

Ingber D E 1993 The riddle of morphogenesis: a question of solution chemistry or molecular cell engineering? Cell 75:1249–1252

Kaptchuk TJ 1983 The web that has no weaver: understanding chinese medicine. Congdon & Weed, New York

Krawczyk WS, Wilgram GF 1973 Hemidesmosome and desmosome morphogenesis during epidermal wound healing. Journal of Ultrastructure Research 45:93

Ling GN 1992 A revolution in the physiology of the living cell. Krieger Publishing Company, Malabar, FL

MacGinitie LA 1995 Streaming and piezoelectric potentials in connective tissues. In: Blank M (ed) Electromagnetic fields: biological interactions and mechanisms. Advances in Chemistry Series 250. American Chemical Society, Washington DC, ch 8, pp. 125–142

Oschman JL 1981 The connective tissue and myofascial systems. In: readings on the scientific basis of bodywork, energetic, and movement therapies. NORA Press, P.O. Box 5101, Dover, NH 03821, USA. E-mail: joschman@aol.com.; web page: www.bodywork-res.com.

Oschman J L 1984 Structure and properties of ground substances. American Zoologist 24(1):199–215

Oschman JL 1989 How the body maintains its shape. Rolf Lines (news magazine for Rolf Institute members) 17(3):27

Oschman JL 1994 A biophysical basis for acupuncture. Proceedings of the First Symposium of the Society for Acupuncture Research, Rockville, MD, Jan 23–24, 1993, published by the Society for Acupuncture Research

Oschman JL 1997 What is healing energy? Part 5: gravity, structure, and emotions. Journal of Bodywork and Movement Therapies 1(5):297–309

Pienta K J, Coffey D S 1991 Cellular harmonic information transfer through a tissue tensegrity-matrix system. Medical Hypotheses 34:88–95

Rasmussen H 1981 Calcium and cAMP as synarchic messengers. John Wiley & Sons, New York

Ratner S 1979 The dynamic state of body proteins. Annals of the New York Academy of Sciences 325:189–209

Rolf IP 1962 Structural integration. Gravity: an unexplored factor in a more human use of human beings. Journal of the Institute for the Comparative Study of History, Philosophy and the Sciences 1:3–20. (Available from the Rolf Institute, Boulder, Colorado. Tel: (1)800-530-8875)

Schoenheimer R 1942 The dynamic state of body consitutents. Harvard University Press, Cambridge, MA

Weiss PA 1965 From cell dynamics to tissue architecture. Presentation at Advanced Study Institute on Structure and Function of Connective and Skeletal Tissue, St. Andrews, Scotland, 1964. Butterworths, London, pp. 256–263

4 The living matrix: five views

Now we look at some discoveries that help explain how energy and information circulate within the living matrix. A far more refined view is emerging that the entire living matrix forms an *electronic* and a *photonic* network. A number of prominent scientists have contributed to this picture. We shall mention the work of several: Albert Szent-Györgyi, Robert O. Becker, Herbert Fröhlich, Donald Ingber, KJ Pienta, and Donald S Coffey.

Albert Szent-Györgyi: electronic conduction

Szent-Györgyi (Fig. 4.1), who received the Nobel Prize in 1937 for his discovery of vitamin C, was certain that the random bumping about of molecules (Fig. 3.1C) was far too slow to explain the speed and subtlety of life. He looked for something that could move about rapidly within the living structure, and focused on electrons, protons, and energy fields.

Szent-Györgyi researched the insoluble scaffoldings that other biochemists routinely discarded. In 1941 he made a remarkable suggestion: the proteins in the body are semiconductors. His statement:

> If a great number of atoms be arranged with regularity in close proximity, as for example in a crystal lattice, single electrons cease to belong to one or two atoms only, and belong instead to the whole system. A great number of molecules may join to form energy continua, along which energy, namely excited electrons, may travel a certain distance.
> (Szent-Györgyi, 1941)

To comprehend the implications of Szent-Györgyi's idea, it is important to understand the nature of semiconductors. Conductors are substances, such as metallic wires, that readily conduct electricity. Insulators are the opposite: they are barriers to the flow of electricity. Semiconductors are between conductors and insulators in terms of their ability to conduct electricity. What is extra-

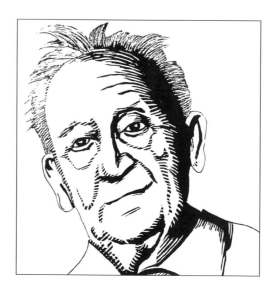

Fig. 4.1 Albert Szent-Györgyi. (Sketch by Arch MacInnes, reproduced with kind permission from the Marine Biological Laboratory.)

ordinary about semiconductors is that their conduction can be precisely controlled. This makes it possible to use semiconductors to make miniature electronic devices, such as switches, amplifiers, detectors, oscillators, rectifiers, and memory devices – the stuff our modern electronic devices and computers are made of.

While Szent-Györgyi's idea of semiconduction in living systems was vigorously opposed, it was eventually shown to be entirely correct. Virtually all of the molecules forming the living matrix are semiconductors.

Szent-Györgyi (1988) also stated that, 'Molecules do not have to touch each other to interact. Energy can flow through ... the electromagnetic field. ... The electromagnetic field, along with water, forms the matrix of life. Water ... can form structures that transmit energy.'

These insightful statements, which have profound therapeutic implications, have been confirmed by recent research. The importance of water cannot be overestimated. Each fiber of the living matrix, both outside and inside cells and nuclei, is surrounded by an organized layer of water that can serve as a separate channel of communication and energy flow. While electrons flow through the fibers (electricity), protons flow through the water layer. This is called 'proticity' (Mitchell 1976). Ho and Knight (1998) have gone into detail about the water system of the body in relation to acupuncture, and have also suggested ways of testing the phenomenon.

While Szent-Györgyi's discoveries and ideas were prophetic of what was to come, they were definitely out of step with the mainstream, and were not given the attention they deserved.

Robert O. Becker: the perineural control system

In a series of important articles, Robert O. Becker described the properties of the connective tissue layer surrounding the nervous system, called the perineurium. Every nerve fiber in the body, down to its finest terminations, is completely encased in perineural cells of one type or another. Becker recognized a 'dual nervous system' composed of the classical digital (all or none) nerve network, the focus of modern neurophysiology, and the evolutionarily more ancient perineural system, which operates on direct current. The perineural system is a distinct communication system. It sets up a low voltage current, the current of injury, that controls injury repair. Oscillations of the direct current field, called brain waves, direct the overall operation of the nervous system, and may regulate consciousness. We return to this subject in Chapters 7 and 15.

One of Becker's important discoveries is that the perineural system is sensitive to magnetic fields. The basis for this research is a magnetic phenomenon known as 'the transverse Hall effect', which indicates that semiconduction is taking place. This discovery simultaneously confirmed Szent-Györgyi's suggestion of semiconduction in the living matrix, and gave a basis for the use of magnets and biomagnetic fields in healing (Becker 1990, 1991; Oschman & Oschman 1995). Becker concluded that the acupuncture points and meridians are input channels for the system that regulates tissue repair. Oschman (1994) suggested that the points may be analogous to microprocessors located at nodes in a computer network.

Herbert Fröhlich: biological coherence

Another area of research complements the work of Szent-Györgyi and Becker. Biophysicists have discovered in living matter a profoundly important vibratory phenomenon that further opens acupuncture and other energy therapies to academic inquiry.

The individual most closely associated with the recent advances is Herbert Fröhlich (Fröhlich 1988). To make Fröhlich's discoveries more accessible to the non-scientist, Oschman & Oschman (1994) have published a review and commentary summarizing this work and relating the concepts to complementary therapies.

In the late 1960s, Fröhlich predicted, on the basis of quantum physics, that the living matrix must produce coherent or laser-like oscillations (Fröhlich 1968). His prediction was confirmed in a number of laboratories. Of course, energy therapists of many schools have always recognized the importance of vibratory phenomena (including light) in healing, but academic molecular science was focused on other matters.

From the work of Fröhlich and others, we now know that all parts of the living matrix set up vibrations that move about within the organism, and that are radiated into the environment. These vibrations or oscillations occur at many different frequencies, including visible and near visible light frequencies. These are not subtle phenomena; they are large, or even gigantic, in scale. Moreover, their effects are not trivial, because living matter is highly organized and exceedingly sensitive to the information conveyed by coherent signals.

Coherent vibrations recognize no boundaries, at the surface of a molecule, cell, or organism – they are collective or cooperative properties of the entire being. As such, they are likely to serve as signals that integrate processes, such as growth, injury repair, defense and the functioning of the organism as a whole. Each molecule, cell, tissue and organ has an ideal resonant frequency that coordinates its activities. By manipulating and balancing the vibratory circuits, complementary therapists are able to directly influence the body's systemic defense and repair mechanisms.

Donald Ingber

Donald Ingber has contributed importantly to our understandings of solid state biochemistry. His work has involved showing how tissue, cellular, and nuclear architecture can be described as tensegrity systems (Fig. 4.2). In collaboration with others, the experiment described in Figure 4.3 showed that the cytoskeleton behaves like a tensegrity structure (Heidemann 1993).

Tensegrity is a useful architectural and energetic concept developed by R. Buckminster Fuller (see Pugh 1976). Tensegrity concepts underlie geodesic domes, tents, sailing vessels, and various stick-and-wire sculptures, toy models, and cranes (Fig. 4.4B). Tensegrity also provides a valuable perspective for ther-

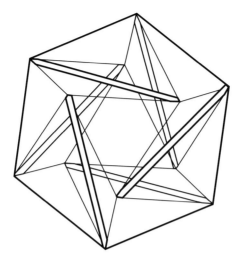

Fig. 4.2 The cell, held together by tensegrity. (After Levine 1985, with kind permission from Johns Hopkins Magazine.)

apists who work with the body from a structural, movement, biomechanical, or solid-state perspective. We return to this subject in Chapter 11.

A tensegrity system is characterized by a continuous tensional network (tendons) supported by a discontinuous set of compressive elements (struts). One might be inclined to place bones in the strut category, but this would be incorrect. For bones contain both compressive and tensile fibres, and are therefore tensegrity systems unto themselves (Fig. 4.4A). Attach tendons and muscles to the bones, and one has a three dimensional tensegrity network that supports and moves the body (Fig. 4.5).

Ingber and his colleagues have brought both tensegrity and solid state biochemistry concepts into biomedicine by describing how physical forces exerted on tensegrous molecular scaffolds regulate the biochemical pathways involved in determining biological patterns – the 'blueprint' Harold Saxton Burr was seeking (Ingber 1993a, 1993b; Wang et al 1993). This work is important to the therapist because it describes how various kinds of manipulative methods can influence biochemical processes in important ways.

Ingber's work with tensegrity provides a conceptual link between the structural systems and the energy-informational systems we have been discussing. The body as a whole and the various parts, including the interiors of all cells and nuclei, can be visualized as tensegrity systems (Oschman 1996, 1998; Ingber 1998).

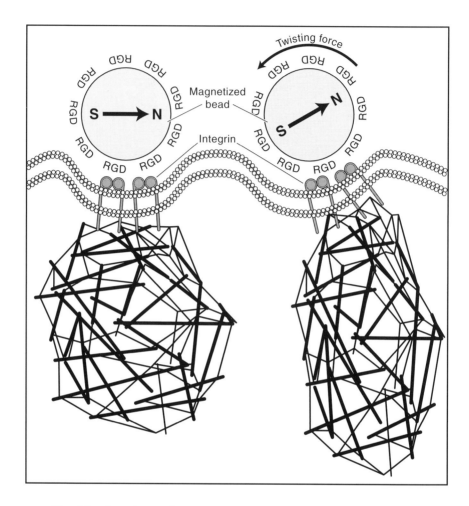

Fig. 4.3 Experiment demonstrating that the cytoskeleton behaves as though it has a tensegrity structure. Magnetic beads are attached to integrins that span the cell surface. The beads twist in a magnetic field, and the relationship between the twisting force and the extent of bead twisting indicates that the cytoskeleton has a tensegrity structure. (From Heidemann 1993, with kind permission from Science and the American Association for the Advancement of Science, and from the artist, Deborah Moulton.)

Tensegrity accounts for the ability of the body to absorb impacts without being damaged. Mechanical energy flows away from a site of impact through the tensegrous living matrix. The more flexible and balanced the network (the better the tensional integrity), the more readily it absorbs shocks and converts them to *information* rather than *damage*.

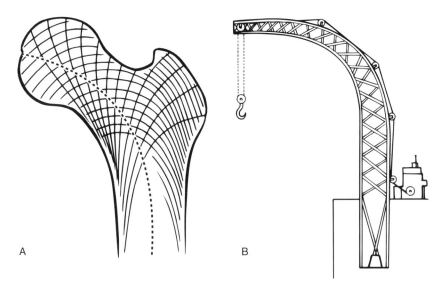

A   B

Fig. 4.4 **A** The head of the femur. **B** A crane. Both are tensegrity structures, as they employ both compression and tension resisting elements to support weight.

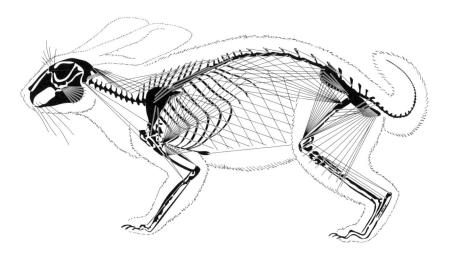

Fig. 4.5 A drawing of a tensegrity system of a rabbit, created by replacing each muscle–tendon unit with a single straight line. (From a figure drawn from life or redrawn from another figure by Miss ER Turlington and Miss JID de Vere in Young JZ 1957 The life of mammals. Oxford University Press, New York, reproduced with permission from Oxford University Press.)

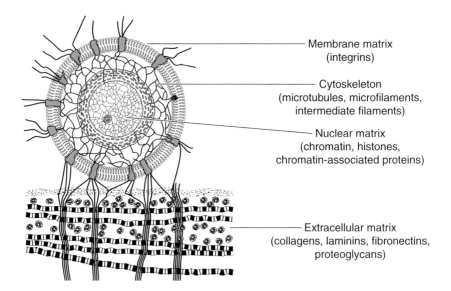

Fig. 4.6 The tissue matrix system as described by Pienta & Coffey 1991 (Reproduced with permission from Medical Hypotheses.)

This concept is useful for practitioners who work with athletes and other performers: flexible and well organized fascia and myofascial relationships enhance performance and reduce the incidence of injuries.

Tensegrity also accounts for the fact that inflexibility or shortening in one tissue influences structure and movement in other parts. While a therapist may focus on improving flexibility and/or mobility of a particular part of the body, the effects can and do, spread to other areas. This is, in part, due to the tensional integrity of the system, but it is also due to the fact that the tensional system is a vibratory continuum. This can be demonstrated with a tensegrity model by plucking one of the tendons. This will cause the entire network to vibrate.

Since the living tensegrity network is simultaneously a mechanical and a vibratory continuum, restrictions in one part have both structural and energetic consequences for the entire organism. Structural integrity, vibratory integrity, and energetic or informational integrity go hand in hand. One cannot influence the structural system without influencing the energetic/informational system, and vice versa. Ingber's work shows how these systems also interdigitate with biochemical pathways.

K.J. Pienta and D.S. Coffey

The ideas presented here are leading to a new image of the way the organism functions in health and disease. The abstract (below) of a 1991 paper by Pienta and Coffey, entitled 'Cellular Harmonic Information Transfer Through a Tissue Tensegrity-matrix System', combines the concepts of the living matrix, vibratory and resonant interactions, cellular and tissue continuity, piezoelectricity, solid state biochemistry, coherence, and tensegrity to paint a picture of the regulation of living systems. Their concept is illustrated in Figure 4.6:

> Cells and intracellular elements are capable of vibrating in a dynamic manner with complex harmonics, the frequency of which can now be measured and analyzed in a quantitative manner by Fourier analysis (and by other methods). Cellular events such as changes in shape, membrane ruffling, motility, and signal transduction occur within spatial and temporal harmonics that have potential regulatory importance. These vibrations can be altered by growth factors and the process of carcinogenesis. It is important to understand the mechanism by which this vibrational information is transferred directly throughout the cell [and throughout the organism]. From these observations we propose that vibrational information is transferred through a tissue tensegrity-matrix which acts as a coupled harmonic oscillator operating as a signal transducing system from the cell periphery to the nucleus and ultimately to the DNA. The vibrational interactions occur through a tissue matrix system consisting of the nuclear matrix, the cytoskeleton, and the extracellular matrix that is poised to couple the biological oscillations of the cell from the peripheral membrane to the DNA through a tensegrity-matrix structure. Tensegrity has been defined as a structural system composed of discontinuous compression elements connected by continuous tension cables, which interact in a dynamic fashion. A tensegrity tissue matrix system allows for specific transfer of information through the cell (and throughout the organism) by direct transmission of vibrational chemomechanical energy through harmonic wave motion. (Pienta & Coffey 1991) (Bracketed additions are author's.)

References

Becker R O 1990 The machine brain and properties of the mind. Subtle Energies 113):79–97

Becker R O 1991 Evidence for a primitive DC electrical analog system controlling brain function. Subtle Energies 2(1):71–88

Fröhlich H 1968 Bose condensation of strongly excited longitudinal electric modes. Physics Letters 26A:402–403

Fröhlich H, ed 1988 Biological coherence and response to external stimuli. Springer Verlag, Berlin

Heidemann SR 1993 A new twist on integrins and the cytoskeleton. Science 260:1080–1081

Ho M-W, Knight DP 1998 The acupuncture system and the liquid crystalline collagen fibers of the connective tissues. American Journal of Chinese Medicine 26(3–4):1–13

Ingber DE 1993a The riddle of morphogenesis: a question of solution chemistry or molecular cell engineering? Cell 75:1249–1252

Ingber DE 1993b Cellular tensegrity: defining new rules of biological design that govern the cytoskeleton. Journal of Cell Science 104:613–627

Ingber DE 1998 The architecture of life. Scientific American 278(1):48–57

Levine J 1985 The man who says yes. Johns Hopkins Magazine Feb/April:36

Mitchell P 1976 Vectorial chemistry and the molecular mechanics of chemiosmotic coupling: power transmission by proticity. Biochemical Society Transactions 4:399–430

Oschman JL 1994 A biophysical basis for acupuncture. Proceedings of the First Symposium of the Committee for Acupuncture Research, CAR, Boston

Oschman JL 1996 The nuclear, cytoskeletal, and extracellular matrices: a continuous communication network. Poster presentation for 'the cytoskeleton: mechanical, physical and biological interactions', a workshop sponsored by the Center for Advanced Studies in the Space Life Science at the Marine Biological Laboratory, Woods Hole, Massachusetts, November 15–17, 1996

Oschman JL, Oschman NH 1994 Book review and commentary [on]: Biological coherence and response to external stimuli, edited by Herbert Fröhlich, published by Springer-Verlag, Berlin, 1988. NORA Press, Dover, NH

Oschman JL, Oschman NH 1995 Physiological and emotional effects of acupuncture needle insertion. Proceedings of the Second Symposium of the Society for Acupuncture Research, held in Washington DC on Sept 17–18, 1994. Society for Acupuncture Research, Boston, MA

Pienta KJ, Coffey DS 1991 Cellular harmonic information transfer through a tissue tensegrity–matrix system. Medical Hypotheses 34:88–95

Pugh A 1976 An introduction to tensegrity. University of California Press, Berkeley, CA

Szent-Györgyi A 1941 Towards a new biochemistry? Science 93:609–611 (Also published in 1941 as: the study of energy levels in biochemistry. Nature 148:157–159)

Szent-Györgyi A 1988 To see what everyone has seen, to think what no one has thought. Biological Bulletin 175:191–240 (This symposium volume contains a complete listing of publications of Szent-Györgyi 1913–1987.)

Wang JY, Butler JP, Ingber DE 1993 Mechanotransduction across the cell surface and through the cytoskeleton. Science 260:1124–1127

Young JZ 1957 The life of mammals. Oxford University Press, New York

5 ▸ Acupuncture and related therapies

Energy flow

Chapter 1 mentions the pioneering work of Harold Saxton Burr, who was convinced that energy fields play vital roles in regulating the structure and function of the body. Much work has been done on the acupuncture meridians, showing that they are low resistance pathways for the flow of electricity (Reichmanis et al 1975).

Viewing the meridians as electrical circuits has led to a number of important clinical methods (e.g. Morton & Dlouhy 1989).

The X-signal system of Manaka

A brilliant overview of biological information theory as it applies to acupuncture has been provided by a leading scientist/acupuncturist, Yoshio Manaka (Manaka et al 1995). The work has significance for all therapeutic approaches. Manaka began to integrate modern scientific research and classical East Asian or Oriental medical theory with a system he refers to as the X-signal system. As a concept, the X-signal system acknowledges that there are unknown aspects of energy and information flow. (The term 'X' is often used in mathematics and physics to represent an unknown quantity. Solving an equation enables one to determine the actual value of the 'X' or unknown.)

In Manaka's X-signal system there are many unknown communication circuits and informational units. A formal mathematical representation of these unknowns is:

$$X_1, X_2, X_3, X_4 \ldots\ldots\ldots X_n$$

Manaka conceptualized the X-signal system to represent a 'primitive' regulatory system that is different from the classical nervous and hormonal systems.

The X-signal system is primitive in the sense that it arose in evolution long before the nervous system. It is present in single-celled animals, which do not have nerves per se, but nonetheless react to external stimuli in order to avoid harm and to attract them to nourishment.

Manaka demonstrated that the X-signal system is separate from the nervous system by describing the various treatments used in Oriental medicine that profoundly affect the body without having any effect on the nervous system.

While primitive in comparison to the nervous/hormonal systems, the X-signal system is extremely important and potent in the human body, as it regulates the communications and cellular migrations involved in defense against disease and wound healing.

In his writings, Manaka presented the X-signal system as a system that is well known from the clinical perspective of Oriental medicine, but that has no scientific basis. However, it is becoming more and more apparent that the energy systems in the living body being documented in this book are all components of Manaka's X-signal system. The energy fields of the body, the perineural system and the living matrix are some of the substrates through which the X-signal system exerts its effects on cells and tissues. The living matrix, the energy fields, the acupuncture meridians, and the various biocircuits that energy therapists interact with during their therapy sessions are all related and are all components of Manaka's system.

Relation to acupuncture

How does all of this fit with the theory of acupuncture? We can now show where the individual cell fits into the meridian scheme that is the basis of acupuncture (Fig. 5.1). The cytoskeleton – which biologists are now referring to as the nervous system of the cell – can be fitted into the scheme. The meridian system, which acupuncture theory visualizes as branching into every part of the organism, can be extended into the interiors of every cell in the body, and even into the nuclei that contain the genetic material. The meridians are simply the main channels or transmission lines in the continuous molecular fabric of the body.

The molecular web is more than a mechanical anatomical structure. It is a continuous vibratory network. As such, it presents possibilities of profound biological and clinical significance.

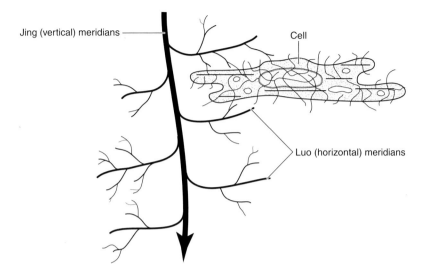

Fig. 5.1 A vertical meridian or channel, and its horizontal branches, which are envisioned to extend into every part of the body, including the surfaces and interiors of every organ, and even into the individual cells and organelles. (Meridian drawing taken from Matsumoto & Birch 1988, used by kind permission of S. Birch and Paradigm Publications, Brookline, MA.)

Hypothesis

Every part of the body, including all of the molecules so thoroughly studied by modern science, as well as the acupuncture meridians of traditional East Asian or Oriental medicine, form a continuously interconnected semiconductor electronic network. Each component of the organism, even the smallest part, is immersed in, and generates, a constant stream of vibratory information. This is information about all of the activities taking place everywhere in the body.

Complete health corresponds to total interconnection. Accumulated physical and/or emotional trauma impair the connections (Oschman & Oschman 1995). When this happens, the body's defense and repair systems become impaired and disease has a chance to take hold. Acupuncture and other energy therapies restore and balance the vibratory circuitry, with obvious and profound benefits. The body's defense and repair systems are able to repair themselves.

Many individuals, both scientists and therapists, have contributed valuable insights to this emerging picture of how the body functions in health and disease. Phenomena that previously seemed disconnected and unrelated are now complementing one another, giving us a more complete understanding than we could have obtained by any single approach.

References

Manaka Y, Itaya K, Birch S 1995 Chasing the dragon's tail: the theory and practice of acupuncture in the work of Yoshio Manaka. Paradigm Publications, Brookline, MA

Matsumoto K, Birch S 1988 Hara diagnosis: reflections on the sea. Paradigm, Brookline, MA, p 142

Morton M A, Dlouhy C 1989 Energy fields in medicine. John E. Fetzer Foundation, Kalamazoo, Ml

Oschman JL, Oschman NH 1995 Physiological and emotional effects of acupuncture needle insertion. Proceedings of the Second Symposium of the Society for Acupuncture Research, SAR, Boston

Reichmanis M, Marino A A, Becker R O 1975 Electrical correlates of acupuncture points. IEEE Transactions on Biomedical Engineering, 22 (November): 533–535

6 ▸ Polarity, therapeutic touch, magnet therapy, and related methods

Let not wisdom scoff at strange notions or isolated facts. Let them be explored. For the strange notion is a new vision and the isolated fact a new clay, possible foundations of tomorrow's science.
Edward F. Adolph (Fregly & Fregly 1982)

After decades of being 'off limits' to academic science and Western medical practice, there is a resurgence of interest in energy medicine. Two areas of research are being extensively investigated: the study of magnetic fields produced by living things – *biomagnetism* – and the study of the effects of magnetic fields on living systems – *magnetobiology*.

Two techniques, representing opposite philosophies, are gaining popularity in hospitals and other clinical settings. The mainstream approach involves the use of artificial electric and magnetic fields to 'jump start' healing processes. The traditional or complementary method is non-contact therapeutic touch, which is increasingly being used by hospital nurses and other practitioners (Quinn 1984, 1992, 1993; Krieger 1975). Closely related 'energy' methods, such as polarity therapy, Reiki, Johrei, aura balancing, magnet therapy, acupuncture, etc., are also gaining in public acceptance.

Modern research is reconciling these superficially divergent approaches, both in terms of their remarkable effectiveness, and in terms of the mechanisms by which they produce their effects. There are good reasons to believe that all the methods mentioned above involve similar cellular and molecular mechanisms.

Medical use of electricity and magnetism

Should you fracture a bone in an arm or leg, and it fails to heal in 3–6 months, there is a good chance that your physician will prescribe an energy method called pulsed electromagnetic field (PEMF) therapy. Your prescription is for a small battery-powered pulse generator (Fig. 6.1A) connected to a coil that you will place next to your injury for 8–10 hours/day. The PEMF device produces a magnetic field that *induces* currents to flow in nearby tissues (Figs 6.1B and 6.1C). Induction is the process by which magnetic fields cause currents to flow in nearby conductors. It is the basis for transformers and other electrical devices. The laws governing induction have been a cornerstone of physics and electrical engineering for well over a century. Clinical tests have proved that PEMF therapy will 'jump start' bone repair. Medical research has revealed that magnetic fields 'can convert a stalled healing process into active repair, even in patients unhealed for as long as 40 years' (Bassett 1995). Hence Western science

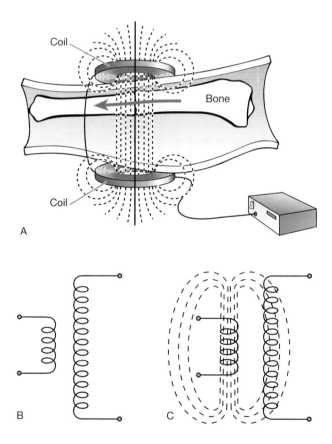

Fig. 6.1 **A** Pulsed magnetic field therapy involves passing currents through coils adjacent to an injury such as a bone fracture. The magnetic fields induce a current flow in the bone (arrow) that 'jump-starts' the healing process (a conclusion of Bassett 1995). **B** A transformer is composed of two coils of wire placed next to each other. **C** Helical flow of electricity through coil on left produces a magnetic field that induces a current flow in the adjacent coil.

has finally confirmed and accepted a concept that has been part of traditional energy medicine for thousands of years.

The idea of jump starting a healing process is familiar to anyone who has practiced energetic bodywork or movement therapies. It is fascinating to follow the saga of how the energetic approach to bone healing was discovered, accepted as a therapy, rejected and reinstated by the medical community.

Modern use of energy fields to stimulate bone repair began shortly after the discovery of 'animal electricity' at the end of the 18th century. By the mid-1800s, the preferred method for treating slow healing fractures was to pass electricity through needles surgically implanted in the fracture region. The technique was banished from medical practice, along with unproven electrotherapies, early in the 1900s (see Ch. 1).

In the 1950s and 1960s, there was a resurgence of medical interest in electric and magnetic therapy. After considerable effort by scientists at a number of research centres (Brighton et al 1981, Bassett et al 1982), both electric and magnetic therapy for fracture 'non-unions' were granted the 'safe and effective' classification by the US Food and Drug Administration (FDA). To obtain this status, many studies were done to document the success, lack of side-effects and mechanisms of energy field methods.

Not surprisingly, the scientific evidence is that PEMF therapy is effective because it conveys 'information' that triggers specific repair activities within the body. The currents induced in tissues by PEMF mimic the natural electrical activities created within bones during movements. Pulsing magnetic fields initiate a cascade of activities, from the cell membrane to the nucleus and on to the gene level, where specific changes take place (Bassett 1955).

Magnetism and soft tissue healing

After several decades of clinical success with the use of electric and magnetic fields to facilitate healing in hard tissues (bone), attention has turned to injuries of soft tissues, such as nerve, skin, muscle, and tendon, and the pain associated with such injuries.

Magnetic fields have advantages over electric fields because they are considered non-invasive, and can be used for treating both soft and hard tissues simultaneously. Each tissue responds to a different frequency of pulsation.

Research employing electric and magnetic fields on soft tissues has been reviewed by Sisken & Walker (1995). The following effects have been observed:

◆ Enhancement of capillary formation

◆ Decreased necrosis

◆ Reduced swelling

◆ Diminished pain

◆ Faster functional recovery

◆ Reduction in depth, area, and pain in skin wounds

◆ Reduced muscle loss after ligament surgery (10 Hz optimum)

◆ Increased tensile strength of ligaments

◆ Acceleration of nerve regeneration and functional recovery.

A fascinating result was obtained in the research on nerve regeneration in rats. In the experiments, the sciatic nerve was damaged, and the entire animal was pulsed with a magnetic field. Nerve regeneration and functional recovery were accelerated. In some experiments, the animals were treated before the nerves were crushed. The pretreatment gave the same stimulation of nerve growth that was observed when the animals were treated after nerve damage. In other words, energy field therapy prior to injury enhanced the body's ability to respond to subsequent injury.

To be effective, PEMF pulses must be of low energy and extremely low frequency (ELF). Recent research shows that comparable fields emanate from the hands of practitioners of therapeutic touch and related methods.

Fields projected from the hands

Chapter 2 documented how the movements of electricity within the human body create biomagnetic fields in the surrounding space. Figure 6.2 shows the shape of the biomagnetic field around the body, as visualized in polarity therapy. There are good reasons (given in the legend to the illustration), to suspect that this is an approximate representation of the overall biomagnetic field of the body, recognizing that there will be local variations in the field related to activities taking place within the various tissues. For example, the inset for Figure 6.2 shows a representation of the detailed structure of the field around the head.

In the early 1980s, Dr John Zimmerman (Fig. 6.3) began a series of important studies on therapeutic touch with a SQUID magnetometer at the University of

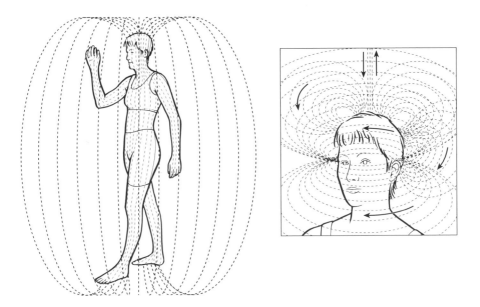

Fig. 6.2 The overall biomagnetic field of the human body as visualized in polarity therapy. Each organ and each tissue contributes to this pattern, which varies from moment to moment in relation to functional activities. The overall shape of the field results mainly from currents set up in the body by the heart, which produces the strongest biomagnetic field. The field is comparable in shape to that developed by the coil shown in Figure 6.1B. It is centred around the body axis because of the helical flow of heart electricity through a variety of tissues. The main flows are through the circulatory system, which is a good conductor because it is filled with a saline solution, plasma (Eyster et al 1933). As with the coil shown in Figure 6.1B, blood flow up and down through the aorta and major arteries is helical. Muscles are also good conductors of electricity, particularly along their longitudinal axes. There is resistance to current flow across the belly of a muscle. The musculature of the heart and arteries all the way down to the pre-capillaries is helically oriented (for references on helical flow and musculature in the circulatory system, see Marinelli et al 1995). As the vascular system begins at the heart and extends into every nook and cranny of the body, it is ideally suited to distribute heart electricity to all of the tissues. (There are about 50 000 miles of blood vessels in the body). In addition, currents set up by the heart flow through the vertically-oriented muscles associated with the vertebral column and backs of the legs – the erectors and hamstring system (Eyster et al 1933). The inset shows a representation of the field around the head in an etching drawn by Edwin D. Babbitt (1896), and is based on the patterns of light he observed around the body after spending some weeks in the dark, which greatly increased his visual sensitivity. Possible mechanisms involved in sensing energy fields will be discussed in later chapters. The pattern drawn by Babbitt corresponds primarily to the biomagnetic field expected from movements of nerve impulses through the corpus callosum connecting the two hemispheres of the brain.

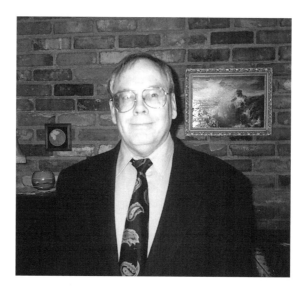

Fig. 6.3 Dr John Zimmerman, reproduced with his permission.

Colorado School of Medicine in Denver (Zimmerman 1990). The experiments were done with a SQUID detector of great sensitivity that had been designed to study some of the weakest of the human biomagnetic fields. These are called evoked fields; they are produced in the space around the head in response to external stimuli such as sounds or visual images (e.g. Reite & Zimmerman 1978).

A therapeutic touch practitioner and his patient entered a magnetically shielded chamber containing a SQUID detector. The practitioner held his hand close to the patient, and a baseline recording was made with the SQUID. Then the therapist relaxed into the meditative or healing state that is the focus of the therapeutic touch method. Immediately the SQUID detected a large biomagnetic field emanating from the practitioner's hand. The field was so strong that the amplifiers and recorder had to be readjusted so that a recording could be made. This was the strongest biomagnetic field Dr Zimmerman had encountered in his years of medical research using the SQUID.

The therapeutic touch signal pulsed at a variable frequency, ranging from 0.3 to 30 Hz, with most of the activity in the range of 7–8 Hz. In other words, the signal emitted by the practitioner is not steady or constant, it 'sweeps' or 'scans' through a range of frequencies. One of the recordings is shown in Figure 6.4.

The pulsations are interesting in relation to the experiences of energy practitioners, who often report a sensation of vibration or tingling during the period when the technique seems to be particularly effective.

In Zimmerman's studies, non-practitioners were unable to produce the biomagnetic pulses. Recording sessions were repeated eight times and strong biomagnetic signals were recorded five times.

Zimmerman's observations represent a profoundly important but preliminary line of investigation into energy medicine. A problem was that the biomagnetic field produced during therapeutic touch was so strong that it was out of the calibrated range of the SQUID magnetometer. This meant that it was not possible to quantify the signal strength.

This difficulty was resolved in a study conducted in Japan: Seto et al (1992) confirmed that an extraordinarily large biomagnetic field emanates from the hands of practitioners of a variety of healing and martial arts techniques, including QiGong, yoga, meditation, Zen, etc. The fields were measured with a simple magnetometer consisting of two 80 000 turn coils and a sensitive amplifier. The fields had a strength of about 10^{-3} gauss, which is about 1000 times stronger than the strongest human biomagnetic fields (from the heart) which are about 10^{-6} gauss and about 1 000 000 times stronger than the fields produced by the brain. Figure 6.5 summarizes the Seto experiment and shows a typical recording. As in Zimmerman's study, the biomagnetic field pulsed with a variable frequency centered around 8–10 Hz.

The work of Zimmerman and Seto and colleagues has profound implications in terms of correlating ancient concepts of energy medicine with modern science. Neither study documented that any clinical healing was taking place during the projection of energy, so further investigation is definitely needed. However, the evidence shows that practitioners can emit powerful pulsing biomagnetic fields in the same frequency range that biomedical researchers

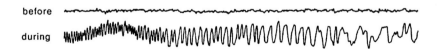

before

during

Fig. 6.4 Biomagnetic recordings made before and during a therapeutic touch session. During the 'healing state' the signal pulsed at a variable frequency, ranging from 0.3 to 30 Hz, with most of the activity in the range 7–8 Hz. (The recordings were made by Dr John Zimmerman at the University of Colorado School of Medicine in Denver and reproduced by Dr Zimmerman's generous permission.)

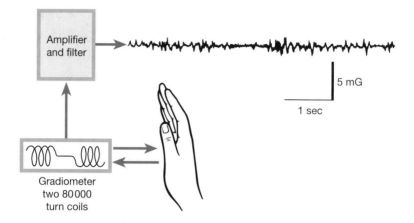

Fig. 6.5 Biomagnetic field measurement during 'Qi emission' from the hand of a female subject in Tokyo. The double-coil magnetometer recorded a pulsating magnetic field that averaged 2 mGauss, peak to peak, with frequency of 8–10 Hz. (After Seto et al 1992, with kind permission from Acupuncture and Electro-Therapeutics Research International Journal and Cognizant Communications Corporation.)

have identified for jump starting healing of soft and hard tissue injuries. This implies that biomagnetism is one form of the elusive Qi energy or life force. The projected fields are so strong that they can be detected with a relatively simple magnetometer, indicating that it is a robust effect that should be easy to study.

If the effect is so robust, why was it not discovered before? The answer is that it was described before. In 1779, Franz Anton Mesmer wrote his famous description of the magnet-like sensation he and his patients experienced while he held his hands near their bodies (Mesmer 1948). When he invited physicians to witness his popular treatments of 'incurable' cases, the response was critical and hostile. Academic antagonism toward 'vitalism' hindered serious investigation of Mesmer's discoveries for more than 200 years. Attitudes are changing because, with a little training and practice, virtually anyone can experience the phenomenon Mesmer described. More and more people are having these experiences because of the increasing popularity of alternative medicine, including energy therapies.

As the biomagnetic field extends some distance from the body surface, the fields of two adjacent organisms will interact with each other. This general effect is illustrated in Figure 6.6A. Likewise, during non-contact therapeutic touch and related methods, as well as during manipulative techniques of all kinds, the biomagnetic field of the therapist will penetrate into the body of the patient. This is shown in Figure 6.6B, in which the lines of force of the biomagnetic field of the arm and hand have been superimposed upon an illustration from Chaitow's book on soft-tissue manipulation (Chaitow 1987).

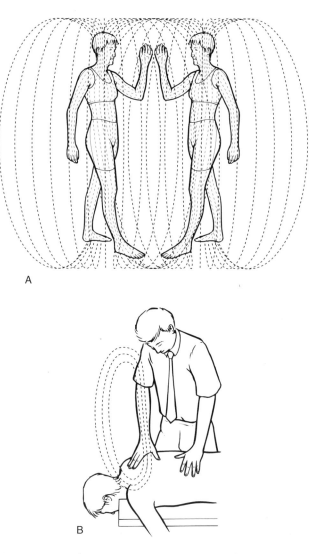

A

B

Fig. 6.6 Biomagnetic field interactions between individuals. **A** The interactions of fields of nearby individuals. **B** Field interactions in the context of 'hands-on' bodywork. Superimposed on a diagram of a soft tissue manipulation (thumb technique) is the pattern of biomagnetic emanations from the practitioner's hands. (After Chaitow 1987, Fig. 13, p. 122, with kind permission from Dr Leon Chaitow.)

Infrared radiations

SQUID research has enhanced our understanding of 'the body magnetic', but this does not mean that biomagnetism is the whole story of healing energy. Several studies have implicated infrared signals (heat) in therapeutic touch (e.g. Schwartz et al 1990, Chien et al 1991). This is important because some practitioners of therapeutic touch and related methods do not experience Mesmer's magnet-like sensation, but rather a sensation of heat or warmth during their work.

Research shows that masters of the QiGong technique can project measurable amounts of heat from their palms (so-called 'facilitating' Qi) that increases cell growth, DNA and protein synthesis, and cell respiration. Practitioners can also produce 'inhibiting' Qi, in which infrared energy is absorbed from the environment. This kind of Qi slows metabolism. References to more recent work on infrared and biomagnetic and QiGong effects can be found in an article from the Mount Sinai School of Medicine in New York (Muehsam et al 1994). A description of healing effects of QiGong can be found in a series of articles published for physicians (Walker 1994).

One explanation for facilitating and inhibiting Qi is based on the fact that the circulation to the skin is influenced by the autonomic nervous system. Years of research into biofeedback shows that anyone can learn to control autonomic parameters, including skin temperature. For example, biofeedback regulation of skin temperature has been used to treat migraine headache. Figure 6.7 shows how changes in circulation alter skin temperature. The rates of chemical reactions and other processes are affected by ambient temperature, so a warm or a cool hand near another person can increase or decrease the rates of temperature-sensitive activities within their bodies.

Some conclusions

In the past, many conventional doctors accepted or at least tolerated therapeutic touch because it seemed harmless, but doubted that the method had any real value. Medical research is changing this picture. We now know that the various energy therapies, including both complementary methods and those approved for medical practice (PEMF devices), have many similarities in terms of their effectiveness in stimulating tissue healing, and in terms of the mechanisms by which they influence tissues. A common denominator is the production of pulsating magnetic fields that induce currents to flow within tissues. Infrared energy (heat) and other forms of energy are probably involved as well. As

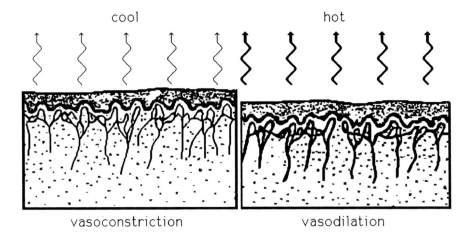

cool   hot

vasoconstriction   vasodilation

Fig. 6.7 'Facilitating' and 'inhibiting' Qi may be produced by changes in the circulation to the skin mediated by the autonomic nervous system. Changes in circulation alter skin temperature. The rates of chemical reactions are proportional to ambient temperature, so a warm or a cool hand near another person can increase or decrease the rates of temperature-sensitive reactions within their bodies. (Modified from Mackean 1973, with kind permission from D.G. Mackean.)

similar cellular and molecular mechanisms appear to be involved, the extensive research on the effectiveness and safety of PEMF devices, non-contact therapeutic touch, acupuncture (see Eskinazi 1996) and a variety of other energy methods tend to support each other.

It is fascinating that practitioners of therapeutic touch and related methods produce strong biomagnetic fields that are not steady in frequency. The emitted field appears to sweep or scan through a variety of frequencies in the ELF range (see Figs 6.4 and 6.5). This is the same range of frequencies that biomedical researchers are finding effective for jump starting healing in a variety of soft and hard tissues. In later chapters we will examine the mechanisms involved in the production of these magnetic fields, and the ways they affect the body. We will also explore the possible mechanisms by which practitioners are able to sense biomagnetic fields.

References

Babbitt E D 1896 The principles of light and color. Self-published, East Orange, NJ [Reprinted several times, e.g. Sun Publishing, New Mexico, 1992; Citadel Press, Seacaucus, NJ, 1967]

Bassett C A L 1995 Bioelectromagnetics in the service of medicine. In: Blank M (ed) Electromagnetic fields: biological interactions and mechanisms. Advances in Chemistry Series 250. American

Chemical Society, Washington DC, pp 261–275

Bassett C A L, Mitchell S N, Gaston S R 1982 Pulsing electromagnetic field treatment in ununited fractures and failed arthrodeses. Journal of the American Medical Association 247:623–628

Brighton C T, Black J, Friedenberg ZB, Esterhai J L, Connolly J F 1981 A multicenter study of the treatment of non-union with constant direct current. Journal of Bone and Joint Surgery (America) 63A:1–13

Chaitow L 1987 Soft-tissue manipulation. Thorsons, Wellingborough, UK

Chien C-H, Tsuei J J, Lee S C, Huang Y-C, Wei Y-H 1991 Effect of emitted bioenergy on biochemical functions of cells. American Journal of Chinese Medicine 19:285–292

Eskinazi D P (ed) 1996 NIH Technology assessment workshop on alternative medicine: acupuncture. Journal of Alternative and Complementary Medicine 2:1–256

Eyster J A E, Maresh F, Krasno M R 1933 The nature of the electric field around the heart. American Journal of Physiology 106:574–588

Fregly M J, Fregly M S 1982 Edward F. Adolph. Physiologist 25(1):1

Krieger D 1975 Therapeutic touch: the imprimatur of nursing. American Journal of Nursing 5:784–787

Mackean D G 1973 Introduction to Biology. John Murray, London

Marinelli R, van der Fürst B, Zee H, McGinn A, Marinelli W 1995 The heart is not a pump: a refutation of the pressure propulsion premise of heart function. Frontier Perspectives 5:15–24

Mesmer A 1948 Mesmerism: with an introduction by Gilbert Frankau. Macdonald, London [This is Mesmer's Memoir of 1779.]

Muehsam D J, Markov M S, Muehsam P A, Pilla A A, Shen R, Wu Y 1994 Effects of Qigong on cell-free myosin phosphorylation: preliminary experiments. Subtle Energies 5:93–108

Quinn J F 1984 Therapeutic touch as energy exchange: testing the theory. Advances in Nursing Science 6:42–49

Quinn J F 1992 The senior's therapeutic touch education program. Holistic Nurse Practitioner 7:32–37

Quinn J F 1993 Psychoimmunologic effects of therapeutic touch on practitioners and recently bereaved recipients: a pilot study. Advances in Nursing Science 15:13–26

Reite M, Zimmerman J 1978 Magnetic phenomena of the central nervous system. Annual Review of Biophysics and Bioengineering 7:167–188

Schwartz S A, DeMattei R J, Brame K G, Spottiswoode S J P 1990 Infrared spectra alteration in water proximate to the palms of therapeutic practitioners. Subtle Energies 1:43–72

Seto A, Kusaka C, Nakazato S et al 1992 Detection of extraordinary large bio-magnetic field strength from human hand. Acupuncture and Electro-Therapeutics Research International Journal 17:75–94

Sisken B F, Walker J 1995 Therapeutic aspects of electromagnetic fields for soft-tissue healing. In: Blank M (ed) Electromagnetic fields: biological interactions and mechanisms. Advances in Chemistry Series 250. American Chemical Society, Washington DC, pp 277–285

Walker M 1994 The healing powers of QiGong (Chi Kung) in 4 parts. Townsend Letter for Doctors, January, February/March, April and May issues

Zimmerman J 1990 Laying-on-of-hands healing and therapeutic touch: a testable theory. BEMI Currents, Journal of the Bio-Electro-Magnetics Institute 2:8–17 [Available from Dr John Zimmerman, 2490 West Moana Lane, Reno, Nevada 89509-3936, USA.] [Also see an article published in 1985: New technologies detect effects of healing hands. Brain/Mind Bulletin 10(September 30):3]

7 Silent pulses

Introduction

At all levels, nature is a composite of rhythms. The vast cycles of the heavens represent an extreme of virtually unimaginable scale, with times measured in light-years. At the other limit are the minute oscillations of atoms and sub-atomic particles, vibrations of trillions of times per second. Life is immersed in this spectrum, and contributes its own unique set of rhythms. One long cycle is that between birth and death. Superimposed upon that rhythm are many cycles of replacement of the atoms comprising the body (Schoenheimer 1942). Some tissues, such as bone and fascia, are completely replaced some 10–15 times during a lifetime, while others, such as skin and intestine, are replaced 10 000 times during the same period. Certain enzymes last only a few seconds before they are renewed (Ratner 1979). Each organ has its own set of activity rhythms, such as the ovary, with its monthly cycle. Shorter yet are the rhythms of the cranio/sacral pulse, the breath, the heartbeat, and the brain waves, which average about one tenth of a second in duration. Even shorter are the vibrations of molecules, which spin, wiggle and shake millions of times each second (see Ch. 9).

Our intellectual history shows a continuing fascination with the ways life is tied to the rhythms of nature, including the earliest astrological speculations, which far antedate the modern science of astronomy. Recent scientific explorations have replaced many early superstitions with accurate and repeatable observations and measurements. This exploration has had a pulse of its own, as ideas of one generation give way to new truths, based on new data.

We shall see that the exploration of biological rhythms has been confusing and controversial. There is an appropriate scientific style for presenting this story without adding to the confusion. Instead of listing interpretations and conclusions as facts, about which we can argue, we present a series of hypotheses. These are tentative statements that can be tested and confirmed or refuted through systematic research and experience. We distinguish between findings and interpretations of findings.

In terms of healing, important rhythms have been discovered by medical researchers who are employing magnetic pulses for 'jump starting' the repair of a wide spectrum of tissues and for treating diseases. While a variety of signals are being used, medical interest has especially focused on pulsing magnetic fields of low energy and extremely low frequency (ELF). The ELF range is arbitrarily defined as frequencies below 100 Hz (Miller 1986). Similar frequencies emanate from the hands of practitioners of therapeutic touch and related methods. Moreover, the fields emitted by practitioners are not steady in frequency, but 'sweep' or 'scan' through the range of frequencies that medical researchers are finding effective in facilitating repair of various soft and hard tissues. This is a recent and profoundly exciting correlation. Let us take a closer look.

Frequency windows of specificity

Table 7.1 lists some of the frequencies being tested in medical research laboratories and the types of tissues they affect. These are sometimes called 'frequency windows of specificity'. References to the original reports are given in the review article by Sisken & Walker (1995). In addition, various frequencies are being tested for their effects on specific diseases. Some of these studies can be found in various United States Patents (e.g. Sandyk 1995, Liboff et al 1993).

Figure 7.1 shows a signal recorded by Dr John Zimmerman from the hand of a practitioner of therapeutic touch (Zimmerman 1990). The signal frequency was not steady, but varied from 0.3 to 30 Hz, with most of the activity in the range of 7–8 Hz. Figure 7.1 also shows the portions of the 'sweep' that correspond to some of the clinical results in Table 7.1.

Table 7.1 Healing effects of specific frequencies (frequency windows of specificity) (from Sisken & Walker 1995)

Frequency	Effects
2 Hz	Nerve regeneration, neurite outgrowth from cultured ganglia
7 Hz	Bone growth
10 Hz	Ligament healing
15, 20, and 72 Hz	Decreased skin necrosis, stimulation of capillary formation and fibroblast proliferation
25 and 50 Hz	Synergistic effects with nerve growth factor

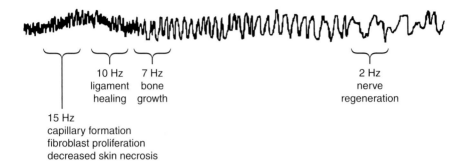

10 Hz   7 Hz
ligament bone
healing growth

2 Hz
nerve
regeneration

15 Hz
capillary formation
fibroblast proliferation
decreased skin necrosis

Fig. 7.1 Signal recorded by Dr John Zimmerman from the hand of a practitioner of therapeutic touch. The frequency was not steady, but varied from 0.3 to 30 Hz, with most of the activity in the range of 7–8 Hz. The second wide brackets show portions of the 'sweep' that approximately correspond to some of the clinical results presented in Table 7.1. (Reproduced with kind permission from Dr Zimmerman.)

Defining 'healing energy'

There is an obvious correlation between biomagnetic emanations from the hands of therapists and the 'frequency windows of specificity' found by bio-medical researchers. While such correlations are exciting, they do not prove anything. More investigation is needed. Research begins with testable hypotheses that can be verified or refuted. We therefore present a hypothesis that is also a definition of healing energy, whether produced by a medical device or projected from the human hand:

> *Definition and hypothesis*
>
> 'Healing energy', whether produced by a medical device or projected from the human body, is energy of a particular frequency or set of frequencies that stimulates the repair of one or more tissues.

Other frequencies are involved

Medical experimentation is not confined to the ELF region of the energy spectrum. Popular devices such as the Diapulse machine emit 27 MHz (27 million pulses per second) and have been studied extensively. Clinical trials of the effects of the Diapulse on injuries have shown reduced swelling, acceleration of wound healing, stimulation of nerve regeneration, reduced pain, and faster functional recovery. References to this literature are given in the review by Sisken & Walker (1995).

The recording shown in Figure 7.1 shows only the ELF portion of the spectrum emitted from the hands of the therapeutic touch healer. Other frequencies and other forms of energy are undoubtedly present. These frequencies can be explained, in part, by the presence of the coherent Fröhlich oscillations mentioned in Chapter 4. For every frequency produced by the body, there are usually harmonics and subharmonics (i.e. signals that are exact multiples or fractions of the 'fundamental' frequency).

The possible involvement of infrared radiation was mentioned in Chapter 6. There is evidence that infrared radiation from the hands of QiGong practitioners can increase cell growth, DNA and protein synthesis, and cell respiration. There is also evidence that living systems emit microwaves (Enander & Larson 1977) and light (Rattemeyer et al 1981, Popp et al 1992).

As an example, the heart produces a variety of types and frequencies of energy that propagate through the circulatory system to every cell in the body (Fig. 7.2). The fastest signal is an electromagnetic pulse (recorded with the electrocardiogram and the magnetocardiogram), followed by the heart sounds, a wave of pressure, and then a temperature change (infrared radiation). Russek & Schwartz (1996) refer to this as a *dynamical energy system*, and describe its potential for communicating information throughout the body.

Mechanisms

Healing of injuries

Medical researchers have stated that energy field therapies are effective because they project 'information' into tissues. This triggers a cascade of activities, from the cell membrane to the nucleus and on to the gene level, where specific changes take place (see Bassett 1995). The interpretation of these findings is that particular repair processes are triggered by the information contained in signals of specific frequencies.

While this is an interesting hypothesis, it leaves unanswered the question of why repair is not activated naturally. Why should it be necessary to trigger healing with an external signal, and precisely how does this signal trigger healing? The following describes some additional considerations.

The living matrix is one medium through which the cascade of activities takes place. Complete health corresponds to total interconnection through this matrix and its associated layers of water.

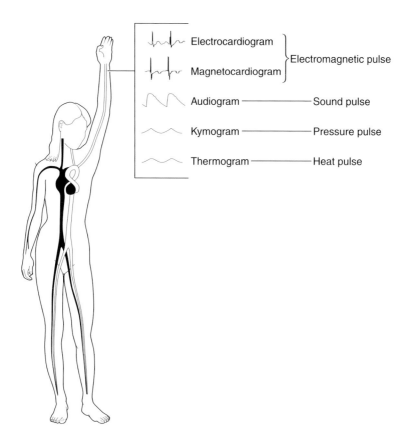

Fig. 7.2 Heart pulses in the order of their velocities. The fastest signal is an electromagnetic pulse (recorded with the electrocardiogram and the magnetocardiogram), followed by a sound pulse, a pressure pulse, and then a temperature pulse. (See Russek & Schwartz 1996.)

Suppose accumulated physical and/or emotional injury or trauma impairs continuity. The application of healing energy, whether from a medical device or from the hands of an energy therapist, would then open the network to the flow of energy and information. Once the whole network is functioning, natural biological communications could flow freely through the entire system, from the extracellular matrix, across the cell membrane, through the cytoskeleton, to the nucleus and on to the gene level, and in the opposite direction as well (Oschman 1993, Oschman & Oschman 1994). In other words, activation of specific processes goes hand in hand with opening of the channels for the flow of energy and information.

A leading medical researcher has confirmed what alternative practitioners observe frequently: application of therapeutic energy fields 'can convert a stalled healing process into active repair, even in patients unhealed for as long as 40 years' (Bassett 1995). The mechanism by which active repair is initiated probably involves both activation of specific cellular activities *and* the opening of the channels or circuitry for the natural biological communications required for initiating and coordinating injury repair.

The free flow of messages through tissues is essential for prevention and for simply 'feeling well.' An example of experimental evidence for preventive effects was given in Chapter 6. Animals treated with magnetic fields *prior* to nerve injury experienced the same acceleration of nerve growth as animals treated *after* injury.

Prevention

While the focus in this discussion is on the healing of wounds, energetic body-work can be of profound significance to the organism even if no specific problem is present. A healthy individual will be both happier and less likely to have an injury or disease. If problems do arise, they will recover more rapidly. Likewise, athletic, artistic, and intellectual performance is enhanced when all of the body's communication channels are open and balanced. This point is well understood in many complementary practices, in which regular maintenance treatments or 'tune-ups' are given. These treatments are not for specific ailments, but serve to reduce the future incidence of medical problems, to enhance performance of all kinds of activities, and generally to facilitate the progress of individuals in their personal evolution, or in the achievement of their personal goals or 'destiny'.

One mechanism of prevention comes from study of some of the effects of acupuncture: mild stimulation of tissues (as by insertion of an acupuncture needle, acupressure, shiatsu, structural integration, massage, etc.) can *simulate* an injury without actually injuring the tissue. By simulating an injury, the mild stimulus activates the cascade of repair processes through the living matrix. Mild stimulation of key points on a healthy individual is a sort of 'test run' or 'tune-up' of the repair channels (Oschman & Oschman 1994).

Somatic memories

Along with the healing of injuries and prevention is the role energy therapies can have in releasing or resolving long repressed 'somatic memories' associated with trauma and/or abuse (for more detail see Ch. 8).

Implications

If the ideas presented so far are valid, there are a number of obvious implications. First, on a practical level, manufacturers of medical devices might find it worthwhile to test the effects of stimulators that scan through a range of frequencies, rather than produce a single frequency. It would obviously be worthwhile to simply record the natural emissions from the hands of a therapist, and project the recorded signals into injured tissues.

Some research along this line has been done. A device has been developed that projects signals comparable to those produced by a QiGong practitioner (Niu et al 1992, Walker 1994). Interestingly, this device produces an ELF acoustic signal. Literature on this device and on other effects of QiGong can be accessed through a database (QiGong Institute 1995) and a booklet (Lee 1999).

Evolutionary biology leads to an additional interpretation. The evidence presented so far suggests that an ability of organisms to project and respond to healing energy, as defined above, has evolved as a natural design feature of living systems. Our ancestors lived in a world fraught with hazards, but had no hospitals or clinics to help them mend wounds of the flesh. A natural ability of individuals to facilitate injury repair in each other had obvious survival value in the earliest communities. Evolution by natural selection took care of the rest.

> ### Hypothesis
>
> An ability to project and respond to healing energy, as defined above, has evolved as a natural design feature of living systems.
>
> If this hypothesis is valid, it points to a simple conclusion: no medical device, regardless of its sophistication, is likely to achieve the efficacy and safety obtainable by imposing a naturally generated signal to living tissue.

Biological rhythms and wound healing

The next mechanistic questions concern the sources of the oscillating fields emitted by the hands of various energy therapists, and the reason the signals scan or sweep through a range of frequencies. Research has led to detailed and rather remarkable answers to these questions. The focus is on biological rhythms and the ways they are regulated. Injury repair involves a wide spectrum of biological rhythms associated with the replacement of various tissue elements. How can these processes be coordinated? The problem can be stated as follows:

Wound healing is a remarkable and intricate process, involving the integrated and cooperative activities of a variety of systems. Each wound is different, and the body's response must be precisely appropriate if structure and function are to be fully restored. Dynamic interactions take place between local and systemic processes. A wide range of physiological activities are activated, and all must be down-regulated when repair is complete. Some repair processes persist for weeks, or even longer, after an injury.

Until recently, the medical approach has been almost exclusively molecular. Researchers have looked for, and found, a variety of chemicals that influence the repair of tissues. The clotting of blood involves a cascade of reactions involving many different substances. Fibroblast growth factors stimulate division of the cells that lay down collagen, a major structural protein used in healing wounds. Hence healing can be promoted by adding natural growth factors, or genes for those growth factors, directly to a site of injury (e.g. Vogt et al 1994).

It is easy to see how molecules can regulate the rates of cellular processes by activating or inactivating particular metabolic pathways. However, there is something missing from the picture. How can the ebbs and flows of regulatory substances provide a 'blueprint' for the elaborate architecture of cells and tissues and organs?

The blueprint

Harold Saxton Burr was convinced that energy fields provide the blueprint for living systems (Ch. 1). Molecular biology can account for the manufacture of the parts, in appropriate quantities, but the forces exerted by living fields bring those parts together in meaningful ways to produce living structure and function.

The last entry in Table 7.1 supports Burr's hypothesis. Growth factors (molecules) stimulate the growth of nerves, but magnetic pulsations at 25 and 50 Hz *synergize* or enhance the effect. Therefore, another hypothesis:

Hypothesis

A complete description of the assembly and operation and repair of a living system requires an understanding of the regulatory effects of both molecules and of energy fields. The genes govern the manufacture of molecules in appropriate quantities, and patterns of forces exerted by energy fields bring molecules together to produce functional structures.

This point of view was expressed over a century ago by one of the fathers of modern physiology, Claude Bernard (1839): 'The genes create structures, but the genes do not control them; the vital force does not create structures, the vital force directs them.'

In the words of Strohman (1993), the genes are important but not on top – just on tap! Genes are undoubtedly involved at every step of development, and influence all physiological processes, but this does not mean that genes are entirely responsible for establishing order and function at every level.

Modern evidence comes from a wide range of studies on the effects of energy fields on development and regeneration (e.g. Libbin et al 1979; Borgens et al 1981; Jaffe 1981, 1982). A simple hypothesis can account for the beneficial effects of healing energy projected from the hands of one person into the body of another:

Hypothesis

A variety of electrical, electronic, magnetic and other energetic phenomena take place within healthy tissue as a consequence of the communications needed to coordinate cellular activities. The resulting energy fields are radiated from the hands of the healthy individual. Whether caused by physical or emotional trauma, 'the wound that does not heal' is a wound that is not receiving the natural regulatory signals needed to initiate and coordinate repair processes. When healthy tissue is brought close to such a wound, essential information is transferred via the energy field, communication channels open and the healing process is 'jump started'.

Sources of ELF signals

The functioning of the heart, brain, and some other organs result in oscillations in the ELF range of the electromagnetic spectrum. The principal brain wave frequencies are shown in Figure 7.3.

Over the last half century, Robert O. Becker and others have done important research on the role of brain waves in healing. These studies have many implications for bodywork and movement therapies. Becker's work reveals one of the unknowns in the X-signal system of Manaka (see Ch. 4).

Modern neurophysiology focuses primarily on the activity of less than half of the cells in the brain (Becker 1990a, 1991). The 'neuron doctrine' holds that all functions of the nervous system are the result of activities of the neurons. Integration of brain function is therefore regarded as arising from the massive

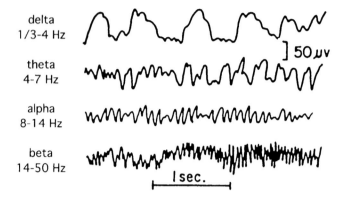

delta
1/3-4 Hz

] 50 μv

theta
4-7 Hz

alpha
8-14 Hz

beta
14-50 Hz

I sec.

Fig. 7.3 Brainwaves. Dominant brainwave frequencies recorded with the electroencephalograph, with electrodes on the scalp. The frequency of brainwaves is constantly changing. Delta activity occurs during deep sleep and in certain brain disorders. Theta activity occurs during various stages of sleep in normal adults and during emotional stresses, including disappointment and frustration. Alpha brainwaves have been associated with a normal and alert state of mind. Beta waves are normally seen over the frontal portions of the brain during intense mental activity. Beta waves of higher frequencies (up to 50 Hz) are associated with intense activation of the nervous system or tension. (After Guyton 1991 with kind permission from WB Saunders Company.)

interconnectivity of the neurons. This view is incomplete because it ignores an evolutionarily more ancient informational system residing in the perineural connective tissue cells that constitute more than half of the cells in the brain. Perineural cells encase every nerve fiber, down to their finest terminations throughout the body.

The perineural system is a direct current communication system reaching to every innervated tissue. The perineural system establishes a 'current of injury' that controls injury repair. Historically, the injury potential was discovered *before* the discovery of resting and action potentials of nerves (Davson 1970). The current of injury is generated at the site of a wound, and continues until repair is complete. One function of the current is to alert the rest of the body to the location and extent of an injury. The current also attracts the mobile skin cells, white blood cells, and fibroblasts that close and heal the wound. Finally, the injury current changes as the tissue heals, and therefore feeds back information on the progress of repair to surrounding tissues. Becker's research demonstrated that the current of injury is not an ionic current, but a semiconductor current that is sensitive to magnetic fields (the Hall effect). Semiconduction takes place in the perineural connective tissue and surrounding parts of the living matrix.

Other tissues in the body are ensheathed in continuous layers of connective tissue: the vascular system is surrounded with perivascular connective tissue; the lymphatic system with perilymphatic connective tissue; the muscular system with myofascia; the bones with the periosteum. Conceptually, the living matrix encompasses all of these connective tissue systems, including the cellular and nuclear scaffolds within them (see also Ch. 15 and Fig. 15.5).

It has been suggested that the current of injury is not confined to the skin, but is a general property of layers of cells, called epithelia (Oschman 1993). If this is so, a current of injury will arise in any tissue, epidermal, vascular, muscular, nervous, or bone, that is injured. Which systems are activated will depend on the depth and severity of the injury. This perspective is leading to a detailed explanation of how the body coordinates its responses to injuries of all kinds.

Oscillations of the brain's direct current field, the brain waves, are not confined to the brain. Instead, they propagate through the circulatory system, which is a good conductor, and along the peripheral nerves, following the perineural system, which reaches into every part of the body that is innervated. Similarly, oscillations of the heart's electrical activity are not confined to the heart muscle, but are propagated through the vascular system, perivascular connective tissue, and living matrix to all parts of the body.

The measurable brain waves arise because of the rhythmic and synchronized spread of direct current through large populations of neurons in the brain. The field is relatively strong and partly coherent because it flows through massive numbers of parallel neurons in the vertically oriented pyramidal portion of the somatosensory cortex (see Kandel & Schwartz 1981).

Becker's research shows that brain waves regulate the overall operation of the nervous system, including the state of consciousness. There is a neurophysiological basis for this concept. The brain waves cause the local fields around individual neurons to vary rhythmically. The local field, in turn, determines the sensitivity of the neurons to stimulation. When the local field is such that the neuron is ready to send a signal (called the threshold for depolarization), a small stimulus will cause the nerve to fire. When the local field is far from the firing level (far from threshold), a much larger stimulus will be needed for the nerve to be excited. Hence there is a rhythm in the excitability of nerve cells throughout the body. Sophisticated research using microelectrodes has confirmed that the probability of a nerve firing in the brain changes rhythmically in relation to the electroencephalogram (Verzeano 1970, Fox 1979). The significance of these phenomena to consciousness will be discussed in the next chapter.

Entrainment

When considering the timing of any biological rhythm, the concept of *entrainment* is important. Physicists use this term to describe a situation in which two rhythms that have nearly the same frequency become coupled to each other, so that both have the same rhythm. Technically, entrainment means the 'mutual phase-locking of two (or more) oscillators'. For example, a number of pendulum clocks mounted on the same wall will eventually entrain, so that all of the pendulums swing in precise synchrony. For this to happen, the pendulums must have about the same period, which is determined by their length. What couples the pendulums are vibrations (elastic or sound waves) conducted through the structure of the wall.

The brain's pacemaker

Brain waves are not constant in frequency, but vary from moment to moment. The 'pacemaker' or 'rhythm section' is located deep in the brain, specifically in the thalamus. The system is known as the thalamic rhythm generator or pacemaker (Andersen & Andersson 1968).

Careful research is determining the cellular basis of the rhythms (Destexhe et al 1993, Wallenstein 1994). Calcium ions slowly leak into single thalamocortical neurons, which oscillate for 1.5–28 seconds, triggering and entraining the brain waves, which spread upward throughout the brain. Eventually the thalamic oscillations cease because of the excess calcium built up in the thalamocortical neurons. During this 'silent phase,' lasting from 5 to 25 seconds, the brain waves are said to 'free-run'. It is probably during this phase that the brain waves are susceptible to entrainment by external fields, as will be discussed below. Eventually the thalamic oscillations begin again, after the cells have restored their calcium levels to the point where they are once again able to oscillate.

The electroencephalographic waves spread not only throughout the brain, but throughout the nervous system (via the perineural system) and into every part of the organism. In this way, the brain waves regulate the overall sensitivity and activity of the entire nervous system (Becker 1990a, l990b).

Entrainment of biological rhythms: more controversy

This chapter is heading toward a discussion of the possibility that external signals, including signals projected from the hands of an energy therapist, can entrain brain waves during the thalamic silent, or free-run period. The reader should be aware that the entrainment of biological rhythms is a subject as controversial among biologists as the mechanism vs vitalism issue discussed in Chapter 1. The controversy is about whether biological rhythms are predominantly timed by 'internal clocks' or by 'external clocks'.

While there are good arguments on either side of this issue, the current consensus among scientists is that biological clocks are mostly set by internal pacemakers, such as the thalamus, and that organisms are, for the most part, independent of natural energy cycles, such as those discussed below. However, the history of science has repeatedly demonstrated that scientific consensuses have a rhythm of their own, as ideas of one generation give way to new truths, based on new data.

Most scientists and non-scientists alike take a firm position on one side or the other of this question. For many, it is obvious that life is part of a larger fabric, and that rhythms of the sun, moon, planets, and other celestial bodies must affect us (see e.g. Leonard 1978). For others it is equally obvious that any such effects, if they do exist, are minimal. For many scientists, there is strong bias against any concept that might be taken as support for astrology, a field that is widely frowned upon. There are good reasons to suspect that a person's point of view on this subject is based less on logical analysis and more on their individual emotional and personality structure. This perspective will be addressed when energetic aspects of personality structure are examined (Ch. 8).

Geomagnetic and geoelectric fields

Evidence will be presented that the 'free-run' periods, when the brain waves are not paced by the thalamus, allow the brain's field to be entrained by external electric and magnetic rhythms, either natural or man-made.

What is the source of natural electric and magnetic rhythms? The magnetic field of the earth, called the geomagnetic field, causes the compass needle to point toward the North Pole. However, if you look carefully at a compass needle with a microscope, you will see that the needle is rarely still – it dances back and forth in a variety of rhythms. Some of these rhythms are diurnal (24 hour), some are much slower, and others are quite fast (in the ELF range). The last are called geomagnetic micropulsations. They are caused by a unique geophysical mechanism known as the Schumann resonance (see also Ch. 13).

In the 1950s, a German atmospheric physicist, W. O. Schumann, suggested that the space between the surface of the earth and the ionosphere should act as a resonant cavity, somewhat like the chamber in a musical instrument (Schumann 1952). Pressing the keys on a wind instrument changes the size of the cavity and therefore changes the frequency of the standing waves within that cavity.

In a musical instrument, tones are generated when the musician blows over an orifice or reed. Energy for the Schumann resonance is provided by lightning. While you may be experiencing calm weather where you are now, there are, on average, about 200 lightning strikes taking place each second, scattered about the planet. To use the physics terminology, lightning *pumps* energy into the earth–ionosphere cavity, and causes it to vibrate or resonate at frequencies in the ELF range (see also Fig. 13.4).

In the 1960s, Schumann's theory was confirmed (Galejs 1972, Balser & Wagner 1960). Lightning creates electromagnetic standing waves that travel around the globe. As electromagnetic waves, the Schumann resonance can be detected either as electric or magnetic micropulsations. The waves are reflected from the ionosphere, back to the earth, back to the ionosphere, etc. (Fig. 7.4). This 'skip' phenomenon has been widely studied, because it is the basis for long distance radio communication. Radio signals of certain frequencies can travel great distances because they are repeatedly reflected by the ionosphere and the earth's surface.

The average frequency of the Schumann resonance is about 7–10 Hz. But when the ionosphere gets higher, the cavity gets larger and the resonant frequency drops. Rhythms of terrestrial and extraterrestrial origin alter the height and other properties of the ionosphere, and thereby alter the Schumann frequency in the range of 1–40 Hz. There are times when solar activity leads to magnetic storms that disrupt the ionosphere, and Schumann resonances cease. Some of the factors influencing the Schumann frequency are given in the legend for Figure 7.4.

To summarize, the Schumann resonance is created by terrestrial activities, and is modified or modulated by extraterrestrial activities. In radio terminology, the signals are frequency modulated (FM).

Evidence for entrainment by external fields

The Schumann oscillations propagate for long distances and readily penetrate through the walls of buildings and into the human body. Schumann frequencies have considerable overlap with biomagnetic fields such as those produced by

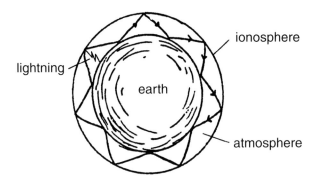

Fig. 7.4 The Schumann resonance is a unique electromagnetic phenomenon created by the sum of the lightning activity around the world. Electromagnetic pulses from lightning travel around the earth, bouncing back and forth between the ionosphere and the earth's surface. At any given point on the earth, the Schumann resonance shows up as electric and magnetic micropulsations in the range of 1–40 Hz. The frequency and strength of the signals depend on the distribution of global thunderstorm activity, local meteorological conditions and the conductivity of the earth's surface at the point of observation. Bursts of Schumann pulses are easier to detect in fair weather, and occur more often during the day than at night. These terrestrial factors are, in turn, influenced by more distant extraterrestrial factors, such as solar and lunar position, sun spots, planetary positions, etc. (See Pressman 1970, Dubrov 1978.) (After Bentov 1976, Fig. 16, p. 145, with kind permission from Integral Publishing.)

the heart and brain, but the Schumann resonance is thousands of times stronger. The similarity of a train of Schumann signals and an alpha brain wave are shown in Figure 7.5.

A number of biologists have concluded that the frequency overlap of Schumann resonances and biological fields is not accidental, but is the culmination of a close interplay between geomagnetic and biomagnetic fields over evolutionary time (e.g. Direnfeld 1983). Hence researchers have examined interactions between external fields and biological rhythms.

Organisms are capable of sensing the intensity, polarity, and direction of the geomagnetic field (Gould 1984). There is evidence that geomagnetic rhythms serve as a time cue in the organization of physiological rhythms (e.g. Wever 1968, Gauguelin 1974, Cremer-Bartels et al 1984), although this continues to be controversial. A variety of behavioral disturbances in the human population are statistically related to disturbances in the earth's electromagnetic field or to man-made interferences:

◆ Friedman et al (1965) documented a relationship between increased geomagnetic activity and the rate of admission of patients to 35 psychiatric facilities.

◆ Venkatraman (1976) and Rajaram & Mitra (1981) reported an association between changes in the geomagnetic field due to magnetic storms and frequency of seizures in epileptic patients.

◆ Perry et al (1981) correlated suicide locations in the West Midlands, England, with high magnetic field strengths due to 50 Hz power lines.

Many studies have demonstrated the probable entrainment of brain waves by external rhythms of natural and artificial origin:

◆ Reiter (1953) measured reaction time, an important factor in traffic safety. Upon entering a cubicle at a traffic exhibition, visitors were asked to press a key. When a light came on, they were to release pressure on the key. Their reaction time (i.e. the time between 'light on' and 'key release') was recorded for many thousands of visitors over a 2-month period. At the same time, the ELF micropulsations (Schumann resonances) were monitored. The micropulsations slow when a thunderstorm is approaching, and Reiter found that the subjects were slower to respond during such periods. When the micropulsations speeded up, into the range of alpha brain wave activity, reaction times were faster.

◆ After the traffic exhibition, Reiter took his test cubicle to the University of Munich and lined the top and bottom with wire mesh connected to an electrical generator. He introduced artificial low level, low frequency signals similar to those

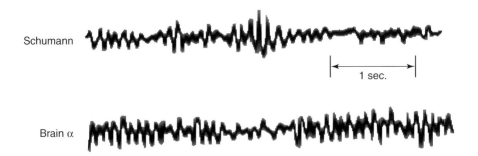

Fig. 7.5 A Schumann signal and an alpha brainwave. After Konig HL 1974a ELF and VLF signal properties: physical characteristics. In: Persinger MA (ed) ELF and VLF electromagnetic field effects. Plenum Press, New York, with permission.

of the earth's field. Under these controlled conditions, the effects of the fields on reaction time were comparable to those obtained during the exhibition. Moreover, subjects in the laboratory experiments repeatedly complained about headaches, tightness in the chest, and sweating of the palms after several minutes of exposure to 3 cycle/second fields. When the headaches faded away, there was often a feeling of fatigue. These symptoms resemble the so-called 'weather sensitivity' complaints that some people have before the arrival of a thunderstorm.

◆ Hamer (1968, 1969) pulsed subjects with low intensity artificial electric fields from metal plates on each side of their heads. Fields of 8–10 Hz speeded up reaction time, while slower oscillations of 2–3 Hz slowed down reaction times significantly. Similar results were reported by Friedman and colleagues in 1967.

◆ In 1977, Beatty reported studies on the practical significance of brain wave entrainment for people such as air traffic controllers, who need to maintain an alert state for long periods. Subjects monitored a simulated radar screen, watching for certain targets to appear. In agreement with the findings of Reiter and Hamer, slower brain waves were correlated with slower reaction times and poorer performance in the task.

◆ Over many years, Wever (1968) and colleagues at the Max Planck Institute in Germany observed hundreds of subjects who lived in two underground rooms that were shielded from external rhythms of light, temperature, sound, pressure, etc. One room also had an electromagnetic shield around it, consisting of a mesh of steel rods and plates that reduced the influence of geomagnetic rhythms by 99%. The rhythms of body temperature, sleep–waking, urinary excretion, and other physiological activities were monitored. All subjects developed longer and irregular or desynchronized or chaotic physiological rhythms. Those in the magnetically shielded room developed significantly longer and more irregular physiological rhythms. In some experiments, artificial electric and magnetic rhythms were pulsed into the shielding. Only one field had any effect: a very weak 10 Hz electric field. This field dramatically restored normal patterns to the biorhythm measurements.

Each of these important but seldom cited studies concluded that biological rhythms can be entrained with natural and artificial ELF electric fields. Entrainment of brain waves can set the overall speed of responsiveness of the nervous system to stimulation. This is called reaction time, and is an easily measured parameter of consciousness. The results support Becker's contention that the pulsing DC electrical system (brain waves) set the tone of the entire nervous system.

These studies do not mean that when a thunderstorm approaches, everyone will get drowsy and react slowly, and accidents will happen. Instead, they suggest that there is a statistically greater chance of slower reactions and more frequent accidents under these conditions. Geomagnetic pulsations do not affect everyone the same way. However, there is evidence that geomagnetic pulsations strongly entrain brain waves during meditation and other practices in which one 'quiets the mind' to allow the 'free-run' periods to be dominated by geophysical rhythms.

Mechanism of entrainment

The internal pathways involved in the body's responses to external magnetic rhythms are shown in Figure 7.6. The pineal gland is the primary magnetoreceptor. Between 20 and 30% of pineal cells are magnetically sensitive. Exposure of animals to magnetic fields of various intensities alters the secretion of melatonin, the electrical properties of pineal cells, and their microscopic structure (reviewed by Sandyk 1995). In addition, various animal tissues contain particles of organic magnetite. Two separate research groups have now recorded magnetically influenced impulses in single neurons connecting magnetite-bearing tissues with the brain (reviewed by Kobayashi & Kirschvink 1995).

The question of whether living systems are sensitive to the earth's magnetic field has been bitterly controversial for more than a century. There are now a number of plausible and well-documented mechanisms for such interactions, and abundant evidence that they take place. Moreover, Becker's research has shown how geomagnetic entrainment of the brain waves can affect the entire nervous system at a very high level of control (i.e. the perineural DC system that extends throughout the body and has roles in regulating injury repair).

In terms of an energetic paradigm for bodywork and movement therapies, there is no need for us to hypothesize that geomagnetic fields, modified by terrestrial and extraterrestrial events, entrain brain waves. Scientists from around the world have already done so, and continue to build solid supporting evidence.

The next chapter explores how these concepts may apply in the therapeutic setting.

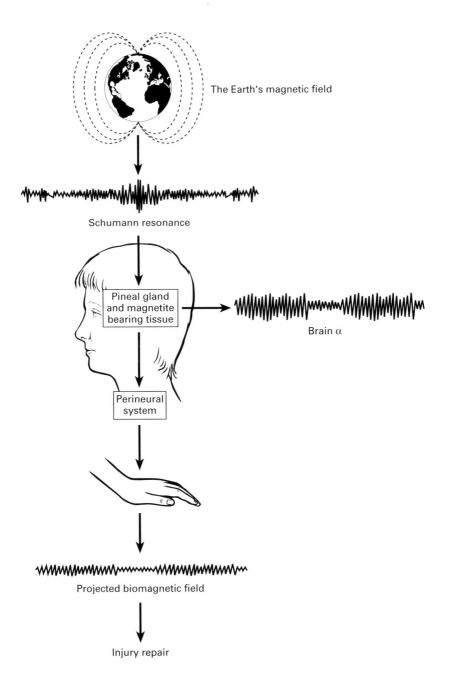

The Earth's magnetic field

Schumann resonance

Pineal gland
and magnetite
bearing tissue

Brain α

Perineural
system

Projected biomagnetic field

Injury repair

Fig. 7.6 A summary of the pathways involved in magnetoreception, the regulation of brain waves and therapeutic emissions from the hands of therapists. Micropulsations of the geomagnetic field, caused by the Schumann resonance, are detected by the pineal and magnetite-bearing tissues associated with the brain. During the 'free-run' period, when the brainwaves are not being entrained by the thalamus, the Schumann resonance can take over as the pacemaker, particularly if the individual is in a relaxed or meditative state (Schumann signals are thousands of times stronger than brainwaves). The brainwaves regulate the overall tone of the nervous system and the state of consciousness. The electrical currents of the brainwaves are conducted throughout the body by the perineural and vascular systems. The biomagnetic field projected from the hands can be much stronger than the brainwaves (Seto et al 1992) indicating that an amplification of at least 1000 times takes place somewhere in the body. Alternatively, the body may simply act as an effective antenna or channel for the Schumann micropulsations. The projected fields scan or sweep through the frequencies medical researchers are finding useful for 'jump-starting' injury repair in a variety of tissues (see Table 7.1). (Portions of this illustration are after Becker 1990b, with kind permission from Robert O. Becker, MD.)

References

Andersen P, Andersson S A 1968 Physiological basis of the alpha rhythm. Appleton-Century Crofts, New York

Balser M, Wagner C A 1960. Observation of earth: ionosphere cavity resonances. Nature 188:4751

Bassett C A L 1995 Bioelectromagnetics in the service of medicine. In: Blank M (ed) Electromagnetic fields: biological interactions and mechanisms. Advances in Chemistry Series 250. American Chemical Society, Washington DC, pp 261–275

Beatty J 1977 Learned regulation of alpha and theta frequency activity in the human electroencephalogram. In: Schwartz G E, Beatty J (eds) Biofeedback: theory and research. Academic Press, New York, pp 351–370

Becker R O 1963 Relationship of geomagnetic environment to human biology. New York State Journal of Medicine 1(August):2215–2219

Becker R O 1990a The machine brain and properties of the mind. Subtle Energies 1:79–87

Becker R O 1990b Cross currents: the perils of electropollution, the promise of electromedicine. Jeremy P Tarcher, Los Angeles, p 80 (Figs 3–4)

Becker R O 1991 Evidence for a primitive DC electrical analog system controlling brain function. Subtle Energies 2:71–88

Bentov I 1976 Micromotion of the body as a factor in the development of the nervous system. In: Sannella L Kundalini: psychosis or transcendence? Integral Publishing, Lower Lake, CA (appendix A)

Bernard C 1839 Des liquides de l'organisme. Baillière, Paris, vol 3

Borgens R B, Roederer E, Cohen M J 1981 Enhanced spinal cord regeneration in lamprey by applied electric fields. Science 213:611–617

Cremer-Bartels G, Krause K, Mitoskas G 1984 Magnetic field of the earth as additional zeitgeber for endogenous rhythms? Naturwissenschaften 71:567–574

Davson H 1970 A textbook of general physiology, 4th edn. Williams and Wilkins, Baltimore, p 559

Destexhe A, Babloyantz A, Sejnowski T J 1993 Ionic mechanisms for intrinsic slow oscillations in thalamic relay neurons. Biophysical Journal 65:1538–1552

Direnfeld L K 1983 The genesis of the EEG and its relation to electromagnetic radiation. Journal of Bioelectricity 2:111–121

Dubrov A P 1978 The geomagnetic field and life: geomagnetobiology. Plenum Press, New York

Enander B, Larson G 1977 Microwave radiometric measurements of the temperature inside a body. Electronic Letter 10:317

Fox S S 1979 Evoked potential, coding, and behavior. In: Schmitt F O (ed) The neurosciences: second study program. Rockefeller University Press, New York, pp 243–259

Friedman H, Becker R O, Bachman C 1963
Geomagnetic parameters and psychiatric
hospital admissions. Nature 200:626–628

Friedman H, Becker R O, Bachman C 1965
Psychiatric ward behaviour and
geophysical parameters. Nature
205:1050–1052

Friedman H, Becker R O, Bachman C 1967
Effect of magnetic fields on reaction
time performance. Nature 213:949–956

Galejs J 1972 Terrestrial propagation of
long electromagnetic waves. Pergamon
Press, Oxford

Gauguelin M 1974 The cosmic clocks.
Avon Books, New York

Gould 1984 Magnetic field sensitivity in
animals. Annual Review of Physiology
46:585–598

Guyton A C 1991 Textbook of medical
biology, 8th edn. W B Saunders,
Philadelphia, PA, fig 59.1, p 662

Hamer J R 1968 Effects of low level, low
frequency electric fields on human time.
Communication and Behavior in
Biology 2(A):217–222

Hamer J R 1969 Effects of low level, low
frequency electric fields on human time
judgment. Fifth International
Biometeorological Congress, Montreux,
Switzerland

Jaffe L F 1981 The role of ionic currents in
establishing developmental pattern.
Philosophical Transactions of the Royal
Society of London B 295:553–566

Jaffe L F 1982 Developmental currents,
voltages, and gradients. In: Subtelny S,
Green PB (eds) Developmental order:
its origin and regulation. Alan R Liss,
New York, pp 183–215

Kandel E R, Schwartz J H 1981 Principles
of neural science. Elsevier/North-
Holland, New York, p 468

Kobayashi A, Kirschvink J L 1995
Magnetoreception and electromagnetic
field effects: sensory perception of the
geomagnetic field in animals and
humans. In Blank M (ed)
Electromagnetic fields: biological
interactions and mechanisms. Advances
in Chemistry Series 250. American
Chemical Society, Washington DC,
pp 367–394

Konig H L 1974a ELF and VLF signal
properties: physical characteristics.
In: Persinger M A (ed) ELF and VLF
electromagnetic field effects. Plenum

Press, New York, pp 9–34

Konig H L 1974b Behavioral changes in
human subjects associated with ELF
electric fields. In: Persinger M A (ed)
ELF and VLF electromagnetic field
effects. Plenum Press, New York,
pp 81–99

Lee R H (ed) 1999 Scientific investigations
into Chinese Qigong. China Healthways
Institute, San Clemente, CA

Leonard G 1978 The silent pulse: a search
for the perfect rhythm that exists in
each of us. Dutton, New York

Libbin R M, Person P, Papierman S, Shah
D, Nevid D, Grob H 1979 Partial
regeneration of the above-elbow
amputated rat forelimb. II: Electrical
and mechanical facilitation. Journal of
Morphology 159:439–452

Liboff A R, MeLeod B R, Smith S D 1993
Method and apparatus for the treatment
of cancer. Patent No. 5,211,622

Miller M W 1986 Extremely low frequency
(ELF) electric fields: experimental work
on biological effects. In: Polk C, Postow
E (eds) CRC handbook of biological
effects of electromagnetic fields. CRC
Press, Boca Raton, FL, pp 139–168

Niu X, Liu G, Yu Z 1992 Secondary
acoustic biological response. In: Lee R H
(ed) Scientific investigations into
Chinese QiGong. China Healthways
Institute, San Clemente, CA

Oschman J L 1993 A biophysical basis for
acupuncture. Proceedings of the First
Symposium of the Society for
Acupuncture Research, Rockville, MD,
23–24 January

Oschman J L, Oschman N H 1994
Physiological and emotional effects of
acupuncture needle insertion.
Proceedings of the Second Symposium
of the Society for Acupuncture Research,
Washington, DC, 17–18 September

Perry F S, Reichmanis M, Marino A,
Becker R O 1981 Environmental power-
frequency magnetic fields and suicide.
Health Physics 41:267–277

Popp F A, Li K H, Gu Q 1992 Recent
advances in biophoton research and its
applications. World Scientific, Singapore

Presman A S 1970 Electromagnetic fields
and life. Plenum Press, New York

QiGong Institute 1995 The QiGong
database is available for Macintosh and
IBM or DOS compatible computers

from the QiGong Institute, East West Academy of Healing Arts, 450 Sutter Street, Suite 2104, San Francisco, CA 94108, USA (Tel/Fax 415-323-1221)

Rajaram M, Mitra S 1981 Correlation between convulsive seizure and geomagnetic activity. Neuroscience Letters 24:187–191

Ratner S 1979 The dynamic state of body proteins. Annals of the New York Academy of Sciences 325:189–209

Rattemeyer M, Popp F A, Nagl W 1981 Evidence of photon emission from DNA in living systems. Naturwissenschaften 68:572–573

Reiter R 1953 Neuere Untersuchungen zum Problem der Wetterabhängigkeit des Menschen. Archiv für Meterologie, Geophysik und Bioclimatologie B4:327 [For a review of Reiter's work in English, see Konig H L 1974b.]

Russek L G, Schwartz G E 1996 Energy cardiology: a dynamical energy systems approach for integrating conventional and alternative medicine. Advances: The Journal of Mind–Body Health 12:4–24

Sandyk R 1995 Treatment of neurological and mental disorders. Patent No. 5,470,846

Schoenheimer R 1942 The dynamic state of body constituents. Harvard University Press, Cambridge, MA

Schumann W O 1952 On the characteristic oscillations of a conducting sphere which is surrounded by an air layer and an ionospheric shell. Zeitschrift fur Naturforschung 7a:149–154 [In German. For a summary of Schumann's research in English, see Konig 1974a.]

Seto A, Kusaka C, Nakazato S et al 1992 Detection of extraordinary large bio-magnetic field strength from human hand. Acupuncture and Electro-Therapeutics Research International Journal 17:75–94

Sisken B F, Walker J 1995 Therapeutic aspects of electromagnetic fields for soft-tissue healing. In: Blank M (ed) Electromagnetic fields: biological interactions and mechanisms. Advances in Chemistry Series 250. American Chemical Society, Washington DC, pp 277–285

Strohman R C 1993 Ancient genomes, wise bodies, unhealthy people: limits of a genetic paradigm in biology and medicine. Perspectives in Biology and Medicine 37:112–145

Venkatraman K 1976 Epilepsy and solar activity: an hypothesis. Neurology (India) 24:1–5

Verzeano M 1970 Evoked responses and network dynamics. In: Whalen R E et al (eds) Neuronal control of behavior. Academic Press, New York, pp 27–54

Vogt P M, Thompson S, Andree C et al 1994 Genetically modified keratinocytes transplanted to wounds reconstitute the epidermis. Proceedings of the National Academy of Sciences of the USA 91:9307–9311

Walker M 1994 The healing powers of QiGong, Part 3. Townsend Letter for Doctors (April):296–303

Wallenstein G V 1994 A model of the electrophysiological properties of nucleus reticularis thalami neurons. Biophysical Journal 66:978–988

Wever R 1968 Einfluss Schwacher Elektro-magnetischer Felder auf die Circadiane Periodik des Menschen. Naturwissenschaften 55:29–32 [In German. For a summary of Wever's work in English, see Wever 1974.]

Wever R 1974 ELF-effects on human circadian rhythms. In: Persinger M A (ed) ELF and VLF electromagnetic field effects. Plenum Press, New York, pp 101–144

Zimmerman J 1990 Laying-on-of-hands healing and therapeutic touch: a testable theory. BEMI Currents. Journal of the Bio-Electro-Magnetics Institute 24:8–17 [Available from Dr John Zimmerman, 2490 West Moana Lane, Reno, Nevada 89509-3936, USA. See also an article published in 1985: New technologies detect effects of healing hands. Brain/Mind Bulletin 10 (September 30):3]

8 ▶ Therapeutic entrainment

Introduction

Evidence has been presented that strong biomagnetic fields are projected from the hands of practitioners of therapeutic touch, QiGong, and other methods. In Chapter 2 it was suggested that repeated practice of various hands-on body-work techniques might increase the size of brain areas devoted to movement and sensitivity of the fingers involved. This, in turn, could enhance the biomagnetic output from those areas of the brain, as it does in those who practice with a stringed instrument. Increases in the strength of the brain waves would lead to a corresponding increase in the output from the fingers, as the brain waves are conducted to the fingers via the perineural and circulatory systems.

Hence the arrangement shown in Figure 8.1 is ideally suited for coupling or entraining the biomagnetic rhythms of therapist and patient. If the therapist relaxes into the state of consciousness typical of those who practice medita-tion, therapeutic touch and QiGong, and other methods, it is likely that his or her brain waves will, from time to time, become entrained with the micropul-sations of the earth's field. If the patient is also relaxed, both therapist and patient may become entrained with the earth's field.

There is remarkable documentation for this concept. In 1969, Robert C. Beck began a decade of research on the brain wave activity of 'healers' from a wide variety of subcultures around the world (Beck 1986). Beck recorded their elec-trical brain waves with an electroencephalograph (EEG). All the healers produced similar brain wave patterns when they were in their 'altered state' and per-forming a 'healing'. Whatever their beliefs and customs were, all healers regis-tered brain wave activity averaging about 7.8–8.0 cycles/second while they were in their 'healing' state. Beck studied exceptional individuals who were famous or who had developed reputations as healers, psychics, shamans or dowsers. He studied a charismatic Christian faith healer, seers, ESP 'readers,' an authentic Hawaiian kahuna, practitioners of wicca, Santeria, radesthesia and

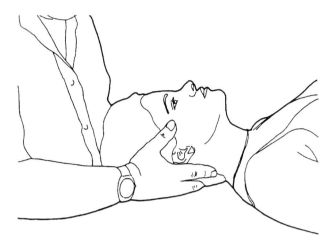

Fig. 8.1 Therapeutic situations such as this are employed in a wide variety of bodywork and movement therapies. Research indicates that this is an ideal arrangement for entrainment of the biological rhythms of patient and therapist. This illustration is from Upledger JE & Vredevoogd JD 1983 Craniosacral Therapy, Eastland Press, P O Box 99749, Seattle, Washington 98199. Copyright 1983. All rights reserved.

radionics. Most of these so-called 'sensitives' entered an altered state of consciousness and produced nearly identical EEG signatures, which lasted from 1 to several seconds.

The obvious question is how did these individuals, unknown to each other and located thousands of miles apart, develop the same brain wave frequency during their 'healings'. Beck noted that, 'the subjects were practicing opposing disciplines, and came from totally disparate teachings, and held opposing viewpoints, and would barely acknowledge the existence or authenticity of practitioners outside their belief systems'. Beck performed additional studies on some of the subjects and found that during the healing moments their brain waves became phase and frequency synchronized with the earth's geoelectric micropulsations – the Schumann resonance.

There is evidence for coupling of both cardiac and brain rhythms between two individuals in the same room, who are sitting quietly, facing each other, with eyes closed, without touching (Russek & Schwartz 1994, 1996). The electrocardiograms and electroencephalograms of both individuals are recorded, and the rhythms are analyzed for the presence of *between-person cardiac–brain synchronization*. Such synchronization is present, and it is enhanced if the subjects are connected electrically, such as by a wire held in the left hand of one person and the right hand of the other.

This approach opens the door to a variety of quantifiable studies of the healer–patient relationships in terms of energy coupling. If there is entrainment of rhythms in two individuals who are not touching, what can we expect from commonly used therapeutic situations such as that shown in Figure 8.1?

Taken together, the research summarized here points to a remarkable model that may explain the unusual emissions of Qi or 'healing energy' and other phenomena observed in a wide variety of energy therapies. What these practices have in common seems to be periodic entrainments of brain waves and whole-body biomagnetic emissions with the Schumann resonances in the earth's atmosphere. The Schumann resonance, in turn, is governed by terrestrial and extraterrestrial rhythms produced by cyclic astronomical activities. The result may be a whole-body collective oscillation, driven partly by the energy of higher frequency Fröhlich oscillations (Ch. 4), entrained with geophysical fields, involving virtually all of the billions of collagen, membrane phospholipid, and contractile protein molecules throughout the body, and, possibly, the associated water molecules. What links brain electrical activity (as measured with the EEG), the biomagnetic emissions from the body (measured with magnetometers), and healing responses is the perineural direct current regulatory system described by R. O. Becker.

If these speculations are correct, the next question is what function coherent biomagnetic emissions would serve in healing. The healing power of projected fields may arise from their ability to entrain similar coherent rhythms in the tissues of a client. Perhaps such entrainment enhances the evolutionarily ancient communication and regulatory systems involved in wound healing and defense. Martial arts techniques appear to involve projecting fields at points in the body's energy system that are sensitive nodes in a solid state informational and power distribution system (Oschman 1993).

The thalamus maintains the rhythms, and the 'free-run' periods allow the brain waves to be entrained by rhythmic micropulsations that are tied to terrestrial and extraterrestrial rhythms. It is during these free-runs that we extract information on rhythms taking place in our environment. Hence it may be necessary to expand our definition of 'information' in the context of healing.

We have seen how medical devices and therapeutic hands-on methods inject 'information' into cells and tissues, and we can now see how some of the information content of these messages may relate to distant activities in the larger environment. An idea of this sort would have been very suspect a few years ago, before the extensive research that has documented the exquisite sensitivity of a wide variety of organisms to environmental energy fields. For example, an important symposium held in 1974 and updated in 1977 (Adey & Bawin 1977) concluded that 'a striking range of biological interactions has been described in experiments where control procedures appear to have been adequately considered'. The existence of biological effects of very weak electromagnetic fields 'suggests an extraordinarily efficient mechanism' for detecting these fields and discriminating them from much higher levels of noise. 'The underlying mechanisms must necessarily involve ever increasing numbers of elements in the sensing system, ordered in particular ways to form a cooperative organization and manifesting similar forms and levels of energy over long distances.'

The studies leading up to this conclusion have been particularly valuable in explaining the ability of animals such as homing pigeons to use geomagnetic fields in their navigation.

Certainly, for those who use their hands to enhance the functioning of their fellow beings, the 'free-run' periods, when allowed to happen without intellectual processing, can give rise to moments of profound insight and deep healing. This is the 'healing state of mind' that is the goal of many healing and religious traditions.

The thalamic relay oscillations resume from time to time. This is important physiologically because there are times when the Schumann resonance stops (as during magnetic storms, when the ionosphere is temporarily disrupted or even vanishes). Therapists often blame themselves for periods when their work seems less effective than usual, when the real 'problem' may be meteorological or astrophysical phenomena that are beyond their control. Therapists also need to be aware of aspects of their local environment, such as the conductivity of subsurface soils, which can be an important factor in the 'reception' of Schumann resonances and other geophysical rhythms (see Ch. 13).

Remarkable as these ideas may seem, they are not new. Deepak Chopra, in his lectures and writings, has interpreted the ancient Vedic scriptures, some of the oldest writings known: 'Healing involves aligning our bodies with the larger body for the effortless flow of information.' Or: 'When my body is completely in tune with the cosmic body, I feel comfortable' (Chopra 1994).

Trauma energetics

This inquiry into energetics becomes far more meaningful when referenced to exciting developments in the therapeutic setting. Pioneers are constantly standing on the shoulders of their teachers, students, and clients, looking beyond familiar territory, scanning for new potentials for methods mastered, taught and practiced. One such pioneer, William Redpath, has, for our mutual benefit, openly and honestly documented his life-long exploration in his book *Trauma energetics: a study of held-energy systems* (Redpath 1994). The following summarizes his journey, partly with his own, well-chosen, words.

Redpath takes us through the evolution and resolution of his own childhood trauma. In the process, he raises thoughtful questions about what lies beneath our traumas and abuses, and the ways they affect our actions and interpretations of how the world works. Because of a professional interest in tragic history, theory and performance, and, later, in various therapies, Redpath shares insights about diverse artistic, dramatic, and therapeutic characterizations of trauma.

His personal trauma was vividly re-experienced 46 years later: the slow motion of his fall, an altered perception of time and space. His teachers (e.g. Peter Levine) cautiously led him back, to face the event, to renegotiate its meaning, to dilute or *titrate* its toxicity. He was guided to look into the dark places, 'where the energy was stored'.

The 'toxicity' cleared slowly and agonizingly as he struggled to emerge from its influence, to reintegrate himself. He recognized that certain behaviours had become addictive, repetitious, toxic, regrettable. Aspects of body, mind, and spirit had been *encapsulated* by the event.

Large shifts, *sea-changes*, unfolded as encapsulating boundaries fell away. Others present at the time of his trauma, who had been experienced as enemies or antagonists, or with fear or anger, were seen with new compassionate, empathetic eyes. In an intuitive and incremental process, his detoxification was rewarded by moments of hope, enlightenment, movement, and freedom, experienced deeply and simultaneously. Developmental processes long on hold were gradually reactivated, with profound consequences for moment-to-moment reality.

Redpath's search was characterized by a remarkable tenacity – from each insight, no matter how carefully and painfully acquired, there arose a set of questions:

◆ Is this all there is?

◆ Is this always so?

◆ If there are exceptions, what do they mean?

- Is it not our lesson to learn how traumas are laid in, how to dissolve them, and how to sustain the resultant freedom?

- Might this be progress?

- Might this be the real source of all of the world's horrors, both individual and collective?

- Might trauma resolution be the only real path to genuine enlightenment?

- Where in our institutions are these vital lessons being taught?

Gradually, through his own struggles and those of his clients, Redpath came to see the mechanism underlying trauma. He saw how his parents passed their own lineage of trauma to him, concluding that the transmission was invisible and choiceless, beyond language and symbol. He realized that held areas represent the body's attempt to limit the damage of overstimulation and challenge.

The trauma of an event is set in place virtually instantaneously, in the fraction of a second before our self-awareness can notice it. Years later, energetic regulatory systems continue to scan this section of held-energy roughly 10 times/second (with each brain wave). Remarkably, stored trauma can be resolved as quickly as it was set in place. The resolution, important as it may be, can happen virtually without notice.

In terms of energetics, one unusual moment of healing stood out for Redpath. A recurring pain had been diagnosed as a duodenal ulcer. In addition to the usual antacids, Redpath began a series of reflexology and bioenergetic sessions, which seemed to help. He learned how to breathe into the place of a pain. One supposed ulcer spasm attracted his close focus and breath, and there was a sudden connection, accompanied by a powerful pulse of energy from the apparent site of his ulcer, up and out of his eyes. It felt like the electrical sensation of putting a finger in a light socket. In an instant, he knew his 'ulcer' would not bother him again, and this proved to be the case. Describing his experience to professional therapists was disconcerting, for they had no capacity to relate to it.

This event was a dramatic revelation of the potential healing forces that resided within himself. The only way he was able to come close to a comparable energetic experience was through acupuncture. (Perhaps his release was actually an energetic discharge along the Stomach or Small Intestine meridians, both of which extend from the abdomen up to the area near the eyes.)

Redpath discerned that our brains are continuously poised to resolve our afflictions, and allow what he calls *serious action*. This is defined as movement that is not referenced to, or motivated by, traumatic patterns, either within ourselves or in the culture around us: 'What if serious action begins not with a movement, but with an immobility, which our brain continuously scans for?'

Redpath found what appeared to be subtle energetic representations of trauma that are readily approachable and resolvable. Because these energetic 'signatures' reside outside the thought and speech centres of the brain, it is easier to unravel them without entering into their narrative representations. This is a definite departure from the methodical analysis of dreams and narratives used in conventional Jungian or Freudian therapies, which do not consistently alter basic patterns. Traditional therapy seeks the memories, ideas, sensations, feelings, thoughts as primary, while Redpath was discovering that there was something prior, preverbal. Moreover, this 'something' could be reached directly, bypassing what lay in between.

He began a new therapeutic style, with those of his Rolfing® clients who were interested in experimenting. Gradually he shifted his focus to victims of sexual and physical abuse. Initially, he worked with his clients lying on the table, clothed. Many are relieved when they learn that they do not have to begin with their 'story'. For the problem is not so much in the facts of the abuse, enormously difficult as they might be, but in the cognitive perception and storage of those facts. Redpath's experience with psychoanalysis was that no matter how well victims recovered critical memories, the patterns of their lives continued to be tormented and disrupted. Where the pattern is most difficult, the brain must figure it out, in the company of someone else but without 'help'.

Redpath's method is simply to place his hands under the base of his client's head and neck (as shown in Fig. 8.1). Over a period of time, sitting quietly with their eyes closed, with some basic guidance, he and his clients watch together as traumas complete themselves. He came to distrust superficial releases, either emotional or physical: they may illuminate without removing the pattern. In contrast to traditional therapies, he suggests that clients not dwell in the emotion. Instead, he asks them to lie still and watch the brain do the work. The work is therefore not physical, or emotional, or willed, or intended. Instead it goes to the deep energetic level that organizes, or incarnates, or underlies experience itself.

In his recent work, Redpath has further simplified the trauma resolution process. Now he simply sits with clients and asks them to draw the shape of the pattern they find when they focus on their brain. Through a systematic process of discussing the image before them, Redpath takes them through the resolution process. He describes the results as a reclaiming of the life force.

Among therapists and others involved, the various perspectives on life force are sources of disagreement. Redpath suggests an underlying reason for this: the trauma mechanism itself causes deep trouble for our brains, which have inherent mechanisms of denial and self-concealment Arguments about mechanisms are another method of maintaining the concealment.

Similarly, there may be a deeper reason for arguments about whether or not an individual's biological rhythms can be entrained by rhythms in the environment, including those of another person. One's stand on this issue may relate more to personality structure and boundary issues than to any intellectual arguments that can be raised.

Microgenetic theory in bodywork and movement therapies

Thanks to the work of Redpath, 'healing energy' and 'trauma energetics' converge. 'Subtle energy' is a concept vast and controversial enough to provide a title to a journal, and to rally therapists of diverse schools. But just what is this subtle energy? If our quest is to be complete, this question must be answered with some precision. We can now begin to do this, thanks in part to a valuable but seldom discussed theory of consciousness that has profound clinical implications.

Rhythmic changes in neuronal sensitivity described in Chapter 7, and Redpath's trauma energetics, can be interpreted in the light of an important concept of consciousness. Jason W. Brown of New York University Medical Center has written extensively on a theory known as *microgenesis* (Brown 1977, 1988, 1991). The theory evolved from careful analysis of certain brain disorders known as *aphasia*.

Microgenesis is a unified theory that brings together language, perception, learning, action (movement), feeling, time awareness, and the nature of the self. As a theory, microgenesis can richly contribute to therapeutic perspectives such as those developed by Redpath. Microgenesis is not discussed widely by neuroscientists, in part because it is based on a wealth of clinical detail that few are familiar with. For example, Brown's work has not been mentioned in any of the articles in the *Journal of Consciousness Research*, which began in 1994.

Microgenesis is a profoundly important theory for complementary medicine, with many practical applications, because it describes the origin of a 'quantum unit' of consciousness in relation to waves of energy (brain waves) flowing upward through the nervous system. The conscious unit is synthesized as a 'bottom-up' unfoldment, a series of steps that retrace the evolution of the brain (see Fig. 8.2). These stages are roughly described as the evolutionarily ancient reptilian brain, the newer paleomammalian or limbic system, and the neomammalian cortex.

Each conscious unit lasts about one tenth of a second, or the duration of a single brain wave. As shown in the previous chapter, the wave begins deep in the brain, in the thalamus, which serves as a clock or 'pacemaker'. From the thalamus the wave of electrical activity spreads upward, into the evolutionarily newer brain structures, ultimately reaching the surface of the cortex, where perceptions and actions come together to form the conscious moment. The wave also spreads outward through the perineural system, to all innervated tissues in the body.

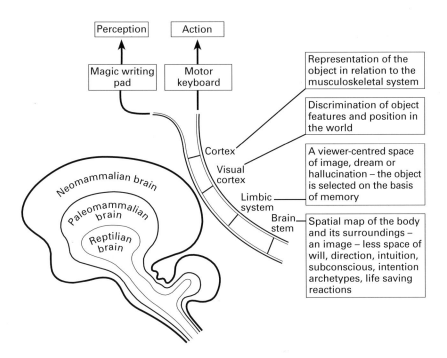

Fig. 8.2 Rhythms in brain fields are related to consciousness in a unified theory called microgenesis (Brown 1977, 1988, 1991).

The neural pathways involved in perception and those involved in controlling actions are linked from the bottom of the microgeny to the top. Hence the brain stem contains a spatial map of the body and its relationship to its surroundings. Brown describes this as an imageless space of will, direction, intuition, subconscious, intention, archetypes, and life-saving defensive reactions. The next level is the limbic system, which is a viewer-centred space of image, dream, or hallucination in which 'objects' are selected on the basis of memory.

In the visual cortex, the features and positions of objects in the world are discriminated. In the cortex, a representation of objects is formed in relation to the musculoskeletal system.

At the top of the microgeny, the conscious moment is written on a 'magic writing pad' on the surface of the cortex. The image gradually fades, from the top down, as a new wave arrives to take its place. The continual replacement of the image on the writing pad occurs so smoothly that consciousness appears to flow seamlessly from instant to instant. At the same time as the conscious moment is perceived, the cortical 'motor keyboard' initiates actions through the musculoskeletal system. Perceptions of the moment and actions upon the environment are integrated at the top of the microgeny.

During the bottom-up process, the 'meaning of the moment' is systematically extracted from a combination of personality structure and sensory information.

As the brain waves radiate toward the periphery of the body, via the perineural system, each wave of sensation references information, both conscious and unconscious, located throughout the body. Sensation therefore enters the microgeny at successive points. However, sensation does *not* provide the building blocks for the construction of the world 'out there'. Instead, sensation constrains or sculpts or selects the developing world from a deep 'preobject', formed from the *personality structure*. Personality structure is defined as the sum of the 'fields' of experience, concepts, memories, and archetypes. Hence the 'meaning' of the moment is extracted *prior* to awareness of the moment. The 'world out there' is what survives a transit through the microgenetic sequence. The result can be a dream, a hallucination, an image, or a perception of real objects in the world.

The personality structure includes Redpath's 'charges', or patterns, or holdings, or encapsulations installed by traumas. It is probably in the lower, preverbal levels, the brain stem and limbic system, that Redpath's subtle energies have some of their effects. Additional effects may be at the level of 'somatic memories' stored in solid state form in non-nervous cells throughout the body (Oschman & Oschman 1994a, 1994b).

It is likely that Brown's fields of experience and Redpath's subtle energies are literal energy fields, microscopic electric and magnetic signatures stored in neural networks and in semiconductor circuits in non-nervous cells throughout the body. It is for this reason that traumatic aspects of personality structure are so approachable when the electromagnetic rhythms of therapist and client are entrained to form a single collectively coherent pulse. By acting energetically, at this silent preverbal level, trauma can be resolved, while bypassing its narrative representations.

The upward unfolding of the unit of consciousness retraces the stages in the evolution of the nervous system, and retraces the ontogeny of the mind (i.e. the development or maturation of the personality). Brown summarized his concept by stating that evolution has taken millions of years to develop the structure of the brain; it takes a few years to refine the personality structure; and it takes a fraction of a second to produce a behavior. Figure 8.2 summarizes the steps in the process.

As a philosophy of mind and practical theory, microgenesis is a *process* model as opposed to a *localization* model. In other words, steps in the processing of data, such as visual information, do not take place in specific locations, but retrace the evolution of the brain's structure.

The microgenetic moment

Microgenesis in action is dramatically demonstrated by those moments many people have experienced when 'time seems to slow down'. For Redpath, this was one of the things he noticed first, when he re-experienced his own trauma 46 years after it occurred: the slow motion of his fall, an altered perception of time and space. This is a frequent recollection of those who have gone through a serious accident or other life threatening situation. The experience of time slowing down is probably caused by a *speeding up* of the thalamic clock or pacemaker, so that each second is divided into more conscious units. While this is perceived as a slowing of time, it is actually a speeding up of the microgeny, allowing for more rapid responsiveness needed to initiate lifesaving actions.

Microgenesis is important for bodywork and movement therapies because it helps account for significant moments of realization, or insight, or resolution that happen occasionally in therapeutic sessions. Redpath described one of these moments, when his supposed ulcer problem resolved in a single instant, probably correlating physiologically with a part of a single brain wave passing through the parts of the microgeny where a certain aspect of his personality structure, a traumatic pattern, was stored. Redpath also described how other therapists were unable to relate to an event so important to his personal evolution. Until microgenesis, there was little in the way of a theoretical framework for discussing such phenomena.

While relatively rare, sudden moments of clarity and resolution are profoundly important, particularly for the victim of trauma of any kind, because they have the potential to quickly and completely re-set the psyche, without getting into the details of the event. A life-changing behavioral transformation, with many physiological and emotional consequences, can take place in a fraction of a second. We can refer to such instantaneous 'healings' as *microgenetic moments* (a term devised by Deane Juhan after careful study of Brown's work). All of this relates to healing energy because the microgenetic moment arises during an individual electromagnetic pulse associated with a single brain wave.

Brown's microgenesis model provides a neurophysiological context for such phenomena, and recent work by Freeman (1995) provides a biological basis. Freeman describes how transient electrical responses to sensation can lead naturally to life-altering changes in the brain. Our interpretations of what a particular pattern or sensation means are set up by experiences we have early in life. Microgenetic moments are instants when these connections are wiped away, leading to a temporary period of cerebral malleability, to new interpretations of reality, and to what Redpath refers to as *serious action*, action unencumbered by traumatic patterns.

Through his own evolutionary process, Redpath developed methods of reaching into the microgeny and bringing about a meltdown or deletion of previously acquired traumatic perspectives. Such moments can lay the neural and energetic groundwork for new interpretations and experiences of self. It is suggested that Redpath's methods represent microgenetic theory in action.

References

Adey WR Bawin SM 1977 Brain interactions with weak electric and magnetic fields. Nash AB (ed) Neurosciences Research Program Bulletin 15(1):1-129 [Based on an NRP Work Session held Nov 10–12, 1974, and updated by participants.]

Beck R 1986 Mood modification with ELF magnetic fields: a preliminary exploration. Archaeus 4:48

Brown J W 1977 Mind, brain, and consciousness: the neuropsychology of cognition. Academic Press, New York

Brown J W 1988 The life of the mind: selected papers. Lawrence Erlbaum, Hillsdale, NJ

Brown J W (ed) 1989 Neuropsychology of visual perception. Lawrence Erlbaum, Hillsdale, NJ

Brown J W 1991 Self and process: brain states and the conscious present. Springer-Verlag, New York

Chopra D 1994 Keynote lecture at Columbia University Dharam Hinduja

Indic Research Center Conference, Health, Science, and the Spirit: Veda and Ayurveda in the Western World, 28–29 October, 1994. [Conference summary by Hartzell JF and Zysk JG 1995 Journal of Alternative and Complementary Medicine 1(3):297–301]

Freeman W J 1995 Societies of brains: a study in the neuroscience of love and hate. Lawrence Erlbaum, Hillsdale, NJ

Oschman J L 1993 A biophysical basis for acupuncture. Proceedings of the First Symposium of the Society for Acupuncture Research, Rockville, MD, 23–24 January

Oschman J L, Oschman N H 1994a Somatic recall. Part I. Soft tissue memory. Massage Therapy Journal 34:36–45, 111–116 [American Massage Therapy Association, Lake Worth, FL]

Oschman J L Oschman N H 1994b Somatic recall. Part II. Soft tissue holography. Massage Therapy Journal 34:66–67, 106–116 [American Massage Therapy Association, Lake Worth, FL]

Redpath W M 1994 Trauma energetics: a study of held-energy systems. Barberry Press, Lexington, MA [Available from Guild for Structural Integration, Boulder, CO; Tel: (1) 800 447 0150]

Russek L G, Schwartz G E 1994 Interpersonal heart–brain registration and the perception of parental love: a 42-year follow-up of the Harvard Mastery of Stress Study. Subtle Energies 5: 195–208

Russek LG, Schwartz GE 1996 Energy cardiology: a dynamical energy systems approach for integrating conventional and alternative medicine. Advances: The Journal of Mind–Body Health 12(4): 4–24

Upledger J E, Vredevoogd J D 1983 Craniosacral therapy. Eastland Press, Chicago, IL, Fig 7.10, p 1100

Vibrational medicines

Introduction

Vibrations underlie virtually every aspect of nature. The vibrations of atoms create sound and heat. Light arises from the vibrations of electrons in an object. When we say something is blue, what is really happening is that light has made the electrons within the object vibrate in a way that causes the emission of blue light (see Weisskopf's 1968 article on how light interacts with matter). At a basic level, all life depends upon molecules interacting through vibrating or oscillating energy fields. Virtually all that we know about living systems is based on the analysis of vibrations.

In the living body, each electron, atom, chemical bond, molecule, cell, tissue, organ (and the body as a whole) has its own vibratory character. Since living structure and function are orderly, biological oscillations are organized in meaningful ways, and they contribute information to a dynamic vibratory network that extends throughout the body and into the space around it. 'Energy medicines' and 'vibrational medicines' seek to understand this continuous energetic matrix, and to interact with it to facilitate healing (Gerber 1988).

The science of vibrations applies to all clinical methods. Regardless of the philosophy of the technique being used, intricate energetic interactions occur between nearby individuals, even if they are not in physical contact. Seeing and talking with another person are energetic interactions, involving light and sound vibrations. Information can be transferred from one organism to another via energy fields, and living systems are very sensitive to them. Add therapeutic intention and touch to the equation, and whole new dimensions of subtle but measurable exchanges are brought into play.

Skeptics lump vibrational medicines together as mystical, supernatural, occult, pseudoscience, flaky, twilight zone, New Age gobbledygook, or, simply, unbelievable (e.g. Barrett & Jarvis 1993, Raso 1995). The dynamic energy systems of the body are dismissed as involving 'subtle energies that are alien to physics'.

These critiques are out of date, as modern researchers have confirmed that living organisms do, indeed, comprise dynamic energy systems involving the same sorts of field phenomena that physicists have been studying for a long time. For example, clinical medicine is beginning to employ oscillating magnetic fields to 'jump start' healing. Vibrational therapies are not magic or superstition: they are based on biology, chemistry and physics.

Vibrational biophysics

Vibrations are a fundamental part of physics. There is a wide spectrum of electromagnetic vibratory frequencies, covering some 90 octaves. Any therapeutic interaction, whether it uses sound, heat, laser beams, herbs, aromas, or movements, involves one or more portions of this energy spectrum.

We have already discussed the extremely low frequencies (ELF) of the brain and heart, and their interactions with geophysical rhythms. Higher frequencies include radio, television, microwaves, infrared, visible light, ultraviolet, X-rays, and gamma rays. For each of these frequencies, vibratory energy comes in discrete packets or quanta, called photons: the higher the frequency of vibration, the more energy per packet. Physicists often refer to all electromagnetic phenomena as 'light' and to their units as 'photons' even though only a small part of the spectrum can be detected with the eye. Biological systems respond in different ways to different parts of the electromagnetic spectrum.

Molecules wiggle

Molecules and their vibrations orchestrate all living processes. Every event taking place within the body involves molecules performing tasks on other molecules. Regardless of technique or philosophy, all healing affects molecules.

No one has ever seen a molecule: they are simply too small. Even the most powerful microscopes give us only a fuzzy outline of molecular shape. In spite of this, we have a detailed knowledge of how molecules are constructed and carry out their functions. How can this be so?

Molecules are composed of atoms, which are made up of electrons. Virtually all of our knowledge about molecules, and about matter in general, has come from studying the ways light interacts with electrons.

Natural frequencies, entrainment, resonance

Previous chapters have discussed how oscillating electric and magnetic fields, such as those produced by the heart and brain of two individuals, can become coupled or entrained, through direct touch (electrical connection), or biomagnetic interactions, or both. We also mentioned important therapeutic applications of entrainment.

Any object has a certain natural or resonant frequency. Strike it, bump it, pluck it, or heat it, and it will tend to vibrate at a specific frequency. This applies to a bone, a piece of wood, a molecule, an electron, or a musical instrument. When two objects have similar natural frequencies, they can interact without touching; their vibrations can become coupled or entrained. For electromagnetic interactions between molecules, the word 'resonance' is used more often than entrainment. In the older literature you will find the term 'sympathetic vibrations'.

In terms of vibrations, the human body can be compared to a symphony orchestra. Each molecule corresponds to a particular instrument. Each bend, rotation, or stretch of a chemical bond has a certain resonant frequency, and will give off certain 'notes' if it is energized. Since molecules, water, and dissolved ions are constantly bumping into each other at body temperature (Fig. 9.1), all parts are constantly jiggling and absorbing and emitting energy.

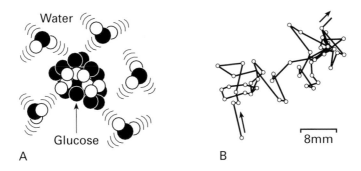

Fig. 9.1 **A** A sugar molecule (glucose) magnified 30 000 000 times, showing how it is jostled by the water molecules around it, drawn at about the same scale. The molecules are represented as 'space-filling' models, in which each atom is drawn as a sphere centred on the nucleus. Each sphere encloses a cloud of electrons. Space-filling models are useful because they show the effective size of the molecule, i.e. the approximate boundary through which other atoms cannot penetrate. **B** At body temperature, a sugar molecule travels more than 3 metres per second, but it does not get far inside a cell because it keeps bumping into water and the other molecules around it. The jagged line represents the path taken by a single glucose molecule in a fraction of a second.

Molecules and energy

While a chemical process, such as the breaking of a bond, may look superficially like a mechanical event, at a deeper level the event is better described as a series of vibratory energetic interactions. This is the level at which the various energy therapies have their effects.

A soprano shatters a crystal goblet by singing a high note coinciding with the natural frequency of the goblet. The atoms in the glass vibrate so strongly that they cannot hold together, and the goblet breaks. The same thing can happen to a molecule. Figure 9.2 shows a molecule of hydrogen peroxide, H_2O_2, being fractured by vibrations. Sometimes this is called 'molecular surgery'.

The O–O bond of hydrogen peroxide is broken selectively with an electromagnetic field of a specific frequency. The wavy arrow in the drawing represents a photon of laser light that energizes the O–H bond (i.e. it makes the bond vibrate violently) just as a tuning fork vibrates when you strike it. The vibrations are

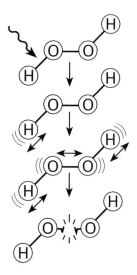

Fig. 9.2 Molecular surgery, in which the O–O bond of hydrogen peroxide, H_2O_2, is broken apart by a specific frequency of laser light. The wavy arrow represents a photon of light that energizes the O–H bond (i.e. it makes it vibrate violently). The vibrations are rapidly redistributed throughout the molecule, and the O–O bond, which is weaker than the O–H bond, breaks. The experiment was done by Fleming and Crim of the University of Wisconsin (see Crim 1990). (Diagram after Ball K 1994 Designing the Molecular World. Copyright © 1994 Princeton University Press with permission.)

rapidly redistributed throughout the molecule, and the O–O bond, which is weaker than the O–H bond, breaks.

'Molecular surgery' of this kind is important to bodywork because it provides a biophysical basis for controversial vibrational therapies in which toxins, such as agent orange or DDT, which have been stored in the body, can be broken apart by energy fields emitted by crystals. When such a complex molecule is 'shattered' by vibrations, its fragments can be detoxified and excreted from the body.

Ball-and-stick images of molecules (such as those shown in Fig. 9.2) create the false impression that the atoms within a molecule are fixed in position. Actually, such drawings show the average structure. In real life, molecules change their shapes extremely rapidly, with time intervals measured in trillionths of a second.

Figure 9.3 shows the basic unit of the protein backbone, called a peptide group. These units are repeated again and again to create proteins of various sizes, shapes, and functions. The carbon–nitrogen bond of the peptide group is rigid, while the adjacent bonds are essentially free to rotate (Pauling 1960). This is important because it explains the flexibility of the protein backbone, which enables proteins to assume different shapes as they carry out their functions.

Computer simulation is used to determine how proteins fold and twist as they perform their functions. The bonds between the atoms are treated as though they are springs. High-speed computers determine the forces acting on the parts. Beginning with the average 'ball-and-stick' structure, the computer calculates the bends and twists taking place from instant to instant as a result of the jiggling of surrounding molecules (Fig. 9.3, inset).

Gilson and colleagues (1994) used computer molecular dynamic simulations to study important neurochemical reactions. They showed how acetylcholine gets to the active site deep within the acetylcholinesterase enzyme. The enzyme has a 'back door' with an electric field that attracts acetylcholine into the active site, and then allows the products of the reaction, choline and acetate, to escape. The process is illustrated on the cover of the 4 March 1994 issue of Science.

Spectroscopy

The most important source of information on molecular behavior is spectroscopy, which is based on the ability of molecules to absorb and emit electromagnetic fields. (For a listing of books and review articles on this important subject, see Sauer 1995.) Spectroscopy is possible because of the resonant interactions taking place in molecules.

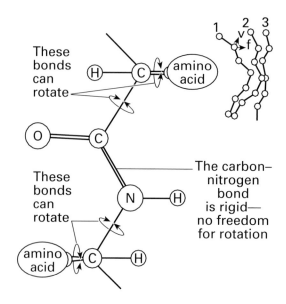

Fig. 9.3 The basic unit of the protein backbone, the peptide group. These units are repeated again and again to create proteins of various sizes, shapes and functions. The C–N bond of the peptide group is rigid, while the adjacent bonds can rotate (see Pauling 1960). Bending and rotation of these bonds allow the protein backbone to assume different shapes. The inset shows three successive shapes of a protein segment, as determined by molecular-dynamics simulation, at 10^{-15}-second intervals. The computer determines shape changes on the basis of forces (f) and velocities (v) created by interactions with surrounding molecules. (Inset after Karplus & McCammon 1986 The dynamics of proteins. Scientific American 254, p. 45, with permission from Scientific American.)

A molecule contains various charged components: protons, electrons, and side groups such as the amino acids shown in Figure 9.3. Each of these charges has an electric field around it. When a charge moves or rotates, the electric field moves or rotates, and this sets up electromagnetic fields that are radiated into the environment. The opposite is also true: specific frequencies in the environment can be absorbed by a molecule, inducing movements of the component parts.

A substance such as water, appearing colourless to the eye, absorbs strongly at a variety of frequencies that we cannot see. We shall see below how such absorptions are involved in homeopathic and related vibrational medicines.

Different kinds of motions taking place within molecules result in the emission or absorption of different types of energy fields as shown in Figure 9.4.

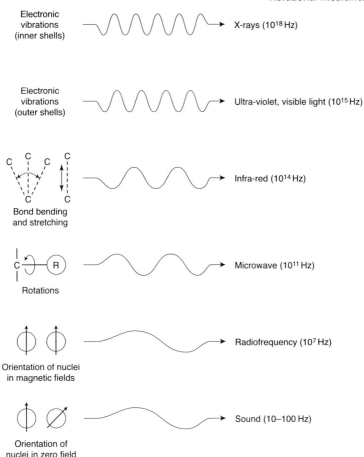

Fig. 9.4 Movements within molecules and the kinds of electromagnetic fields they emit or absorb. The highest frequency and highest energy motions are those of the innermost electrons, which resonate in the X-ray region of the electromagnetic spectrum. The outermost electrons, that are responsible for most of the physical and chemical properties of an atom, resonate at the ultraviolet and visible portions of the spectrum. Bond bending and stretching involves infrared light. Bond rotations resonate at microwave frequencies. The spins and orientations of atomic nuclei correspond to vibrations in the radiofrequency and sound portions of the spectrum. Usually the frequencies absorbed by a molecule are identical with the frequencies emitted when the molecule is excited. This reciprocity of absorption and emission is known as Kirchhoff's principle. Energy is absorbed by the reverse of the process by which emissions are produced, i.e. the absorbed energy causes particular motions to be set up within the molecule. The boundaries between the different frequency regions are not sharply defined. The illustration is a simplification in that it does not show the couplings that take place between different activities, such as between vibrations and rotations. (Modified from Whiffen DH 1966, Fig. 2.1, p 15, by kind permission of Pearson Education Ltd.) For more details see a chart of the electromagnetic spectrum.

Spectrometers of various kinds are used to measure the emissions and absorptions of molecules. Technically the radiation or absorption pattern is called a spectrum (a graph of energy intensity versus frequency or wavelength). Figure 9.5 shows a typical infrared absorption spectrum of a compound. Each peak represents a frequency that is absorbed by bending or stretching of a particular bond within the molecule.

Every molecule in the body, and every homeopathic, herbal, or aromatherapy preparation, vibrates in specific ways and emits a characteristic energy spectrum. Complex molecules contain thousands or even millions of atoms, and their spectra can be quite intricate. The spectrum is an electromagnetic 'signature' or 'fingerprint' of a molecule that is an extremely precise representation of the motions of the particles within it. So characteristic are these fingerprints that a chemist can use them to identify an unknown substance.

Vibratory interactions between molecules

Figure 9.6 shows a resonant interaction between two nearby proteins. The rotation of a charged amino acid sets up an electromagnetic field that entrains rotations of the corresponding amino acid on a second protein. The second protein also emits an electromagnetic field that affects other proteins. As a result, molecular motions and energy fields join together to form a continuous or collective energy system. We shall see below that the crystal-like organization of molecules in living systems enhances this phenomenon.

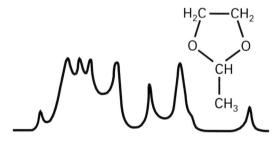

Fig. 9.5 The infrared absorption spectrum of 2-methyl dioxalane, and its molecular structure. (After Whiffen 1966, Fig. 8.2a, p. 102, with permission from Pearson Education Limited.)

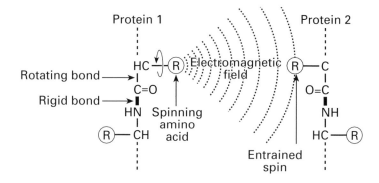

Fig. 9.6 The rotations of a charged portion of the protein molecule on the left set up an electromagnetic field that brings about complementary motions in the protein to the right, even though the two molecules are not touching. It is the oscillating electric component of the electromagnetic field that makes the amino acid of protein 2 oscillate in synchrony with the corresponding amino acid of protein 1. (For details, Allen & Cross 1963, Sauer 1995.)

Living crystals

All therapeutic and scientific approaches to the body can benefit from an appreciation of the crystalline nature of living tissues. We do not usually consider our bodies to be crystalline, because when we think of crystals we usually think of hard materials, like diamond or agate. Living crystals are composed of long, thin, pliable molecules, and are soft and flexible. To be more precise, these are liquid crystals (see e.g. Bouligand 1978).

Crystalline arrangements are the rule and not the exception in living systems. Examples include arrays of phospholipid molecules forming cell membranes and myelin sheaths of nerves, collagen arrays forming connective tissue and fascia, contractile arrays in muscle, arrays of sensory elements in the eye, nose, and ear, arrays of microtubules, microfilaments and other fibrous components of the cytoskeleton in nerves and other kinds of cells, and arrays of chlorophyll molecules in a leaf (see Fig. 3.4, Ch. 13 and Fig. 13.2).

Some bodyworkers are convinced that crystalline materials, such as quartz, shells and stones, enhance the effectiveness of their work (e.g. Jeffery 1993, Galde 1991). A simple explanation for such effects is that crystalline objects have resonant interactions with the highly ordered liquid crystals within the tissues of the therapist and the person being touched. In other words, the crystals enhance vibratory energy exchanges between two individuals.

Coherence

Because of the resonant interactions illustrated in Figure 9.6, nearby molecules interact with each other via electromagnetic fields. What happens in an extensive array of similar molecules, such as those mentioned above?

Answering this question has led to one of the most important discoveries in recent years, a discovery that can help account for many of the remarkable phenomena experienced every day by practitioners of vibrational medicines.

We have repeatedly mentioned the work of Herbert Fröhlich, who predicted that crystalline molecular arrays should vibrate strongly and coherently (see Ch. 4). (For an entertaining account of coherence and its biological significance, see *The Rainbow and the Worm* (Ho 1993).

Fröhlich was particularly impressed with the effects of the enormous electrical fields developed across cell membranes, with the inside negative relative to the outside. Electrical fields are also generated in the collagen arrays in connective tissues (tendons, ligaments, bones, cartilage, fascia) during movements. Activities such as nerve conduction, muscle contraction, and glandular secretion also produce electrical fields. Each activity in the body creates a characteristic field pattern. Moreover, the whole body is polarized, with the head-end negative and the tail- or foot-end positive (Athenstaedt 1974).

Research on electrically polarized molecular arrays reveals that interactions such as those shown in Figure 9.6, repeated by the millions of molecules within a cell membrane, tendon, muscle, bone, nerve cell, or other structure, give rise to huge coherent or laser-like vibrations. The vibrations are collective or cooperative phenomena, in which all of the weakly vibrating parts, in the presence of an electric field, become coupled. The result is a strong, orderly, and stable vibration that is far more than the sum of individual vibrations. This is an example of the tendency for new properties to arise as we go up the ladder of scale, eloquently described by Szent-Györgyi (1963):

> If Nature puts two things together she produces something new with new qualities, which cannot be expressed in terms of qualities of the components. When going from electrons and protons to atoms, from here to molecules, molecular aggregates, etc., up to the cell or the whole animal, at every level we find something new, a new breathtaking vista. Whenever we separate two things, we lose something, something which may have been the most essential feature. (Szent-Györgyi 1963)

Bodywork and movement therapies focus primarily on the 'something new' or 'breathtaking vistas' arising in the body as a consequence of the ways the parts cooperate. In the past, science has been based on separating parts for individual study, which obviously eliminates some of the most interesting properties. Whenever a scientist, such as Fröhlich or Szent-Györgyi, has looked for the cooperative qualities arising from the ways living molecules interact, profoundly important discoveries have emerged.

In the case of Fröhlich oscillations, two 'new qualities' arise that are of great importance in the therapeutic setting. The first is that the crystalline molecular arrays found throughout the body are exceedingly sensitive to energy fields in the environment. Some of these sensitivities border on the limits of what is physically possible. Biologists continue to find such sensitivities, but the phenomena have often been dismissed as impossible. Fröhlich's research has provided a sound biophysical mechanism that can explain such sensitivities. This subject will be taken up again in Chapter 13.

The second new quality is that strong oscillations can travel about within the crystalline network of the body and they can be radiated into the environment. Theory predicted that the vibrations would occur at a variety of frequencies, including visible and near visible light. Such radiations have been detected (e.g. Callahan 1975; Popp et al 1981, 1992). Moreover, it has also been demonstrated that such frequencies have important biological effects (e.g. Grundler et al 1977).

Crystalline components of the living matrix act as coherent molecular 'antennas', radiating and receiving signals. Electronics engineers know that an antenna works best if its length corresponds to the wavelength of the signal being transmitted or received. When a person moves, tensions set up within the fabric of the body change the lengths of the molecular antennas of the myofascial system, and therefore change their resonant frequencies. Experienced bodywork and movement therapists become sensitive to such changes, and use the information to 'tune in' to imbalanced or immobile places within the bodies of their clients.

Research on coherence in biological systems is attracting much attention around the world. One important conclusion is that the water in the spaces between parts of the highly ordered systems is also highly organized. Vibrations of the water molecules can couple to the coherent energy patterns within the protein array. The resulting coherent water system has laser-like properties, and is likely to retain and release electromagnetic information, i.e. have a form of memory (Del Giudice et al 1988, Preparata 1995).

Cellular oscillations and systemic regulations

Now we consider vibrating molecules in the context of whole body or systemic regulations, the focus of many bodywork and movement therapies. Figure 9.7 shows all of the physiological processes in the body, without their names. All the systems are interlinked by a great number of interacting and crisscrossed pathways (Adolph 1979). Systemic, or global, or 'whole system' regulation refers to the sum of all of these communicating pathways interacting and integrating to produce coordinated actions, such as metabolism, movement, thought, excretion, reproduction, defense against disease, wound repair, etc. All schools of bodywork or movement therapy represent different approaches to these regulatory networks.

From the complexity shown in Figure 9.7, we extract a single physiological regulatory loop affecting a single cell (Fig. 9.8). In making this separation, we keep in mind the intricately crisscrossed pathways that operate in the back-

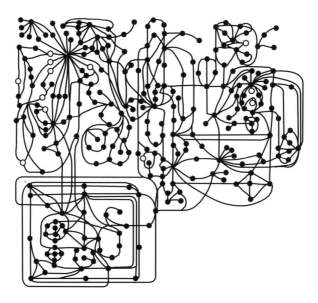

Fig. 9.7 All of the physiological processes in the body are shown without their names. 'The biology of wholeness is the study of the body as an integrated, coordinated, successful system. No parts or properties are uncorrelated, all are demonstrably interlinked. And the links are not single chains, but a great number of crisscrossed pathways. All of the systems interdigitate. This is possible because of communication' (Adolph 1982) (After Mellor 1966.)

ground, affecting every step. We also keep in mind Szent-Györgyi's perspective of the essential features that are lost by making the separation.

The conventional linear way of viewing this scheme is that a stimulus or disturbance to the system initiates a cascade of events that eventually activate a receptor on the surface of a particular cell. Another cascade of events within the cell leads to a certain activity.

An important discovery in relation to this scheme is the existence of 'second messengers' within cells (e.g. Rasmussen 1981). These are substances that convert a 'first' message – such as a hormone, neurotransmitter, growth factor, or other command signal arriving at the cell surface – into a change in some activity inside the cell or nucleus. These events lead to an 'action' that tends to bring the whole system back to balance. A series of signals then feeds back to the first step in the loop, providing information that the action has been completed.

Pharmacology is based on the concept that if we understand a regulatory pathway, we can selectively intervene with drugs that stimulate or block specific steps in the chain. There is more to the story, for each part of the sequence involves a molecule with a unique structure and with a unique pattern of energy emission and absorption. Internal motions of each molecule enable it to carry out its function (e.g. as a hormone, receptor, second messenger, or enzyme). A spectrum of different frequencies will be given off while a molecule is coiling or twisting to carry out its task, and a corresponding set of frequencies can be applied to a molecule that will enhance or inhibit the internal motions involved in the molecule's functioning. For example, a hormone–receptor interaction or an antibody–antigen reaction is often viewed as a mechanical lock-and-key system, in which only one specific type of molecule can fit into the receptor.

While the analogy is useful, there is more to the story of how one molecule recognizes and responds to another. At the atomic scale, physical contact between two molecules has less meaning than the ways they interact energetically. As a hormone approaches a receptor, the electronic structures of both molecules begin to change. Bonds bend, twist, and stretch; parts rotate and wiggle. The orientation and shape of the molecules change so that the active site of the hormone can approach the active site of the receptor. Recognition of a specific hormone by a receptor depends on resonant vibratory interactions, comparable to the interactions of tuning forks (see Ch. 14 and Fig. 14.1).

Fröhlich (1975) developed a model in which strong attractions arise because of giant coherent oscillations of the two molecules involved. The appro-

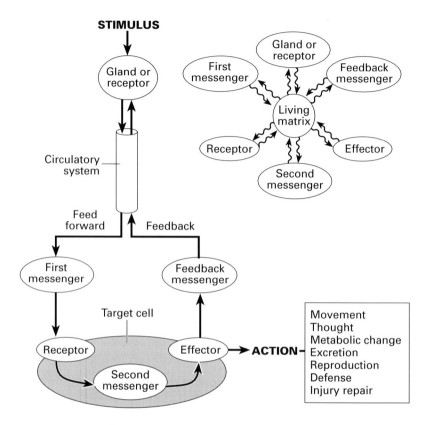

Fig. 9.8 A single regulatory loop is separated out from the web of physiological interactions shown in Figure 9.7. A stimulus or disturbance to the system (technically called a perturbation) affects a gland or sensor. This results in the release of a messenger (hormone, signal molecule, or growth factor) into the circulatory system. The messenger travels to a target cell, where it activates a receptor in the cell membrane. This activates one or more second messengers within the cell that activate an effector (contractile array, secretory system, etc.) causing some action to take place. Feedback is obligatory, as information that an action has taken place always flows back to the beginning of the cycle (Adolph 1979). The feedback messenger enters the circulatory system, and is carried back to the gland or receptor that initiated the cycle. The inset shows that each molecule in the loop emits and absorbs electromagnetic signals (photons, shown as wavy lines) as it carries out its function. These signals can be absorbed and conducted throughout the organism by the continuous living matrix (the connective tissues, cytoskeletons, nuclear matrices, and water associated with them). Some of the components of the loop may be partly or entirely electromagnetic in character. Allergies, chronic and degenerative diseases, and failure to heal can result from the disruption of such regulatory loops. We can view the loop as a cascade of chemical reactions accompanied by a cascade of electronic and electromagnetic interactions.

priate frequency for such attractions is around 10^{13} Hz, which corresponds closely to the frequency of cell membrane electrical oscillations at body temperature.

Activation of the receptor is the final step in an elaborate energetic dance of the electrons within the signal and receptor molecules. This electronic 'ballet' is an example of molecules interacting without touching. As the electronic structure of hormone and receptor changes, photons are emitted and absorbed. Such emissions and adsorptions were once thought to be random events – unimportant by-products of biochemical processes; scientists now see them as vital pieces of information.

The inset in Figure 9.8 shows some of the photons being given off and absorbed by molecules as they perform their functions in a regulatory loop. The information arising from such energetic exchanges is not wasted. Instead, information is exchanged with the living matrix continuum. This is the continuous network composed of connective tissues, cytoskeletons, and nuclear matrices, and the continuous layers of water adhering to them. Since the living matrix extends into every nook and cranny of the body, it forms a systemic energetic continuum. The overall field of the body, and fields in the environment, affect all of the steps in the regulatory loop. Hence the electromagnetic 'environment' of a hormone–receptor interaction influences and is modified by the interaction. In some cases, triggering a receptor with an appropriate electromagnetic field is indistinguishable from triggering it with a hormone or other stimulus. Some important regulatory loops may be partly or entirely electromagnetic in character, and are therefore not recognized by conventional pharmacology. In the future, we can expect chemical pharmacology to be greatly augmented by energetic pharmacology. Fröhlich (1978) explains:

> An assembly of cells, as in a tissue or organ, will have certain collective frequencies that regulate important processes, such as cell division. Normally these control frequencies will be very stable. If, for some reason, a cell shifts its frequency, entraining signals from neighboring cells will tend to reinstall the correct frequency. However, if a sufficient number of cells get out-of-step, the strength of the system's collective vibrations can decrease to the point where stability is lost. Loss of coherence can lead to disease or disorder.
> (Fröhlich 1978)

While pathology may manifest as chemical imbalances, the underlying problem is electromagnetic. Hence balance can often be restored by providing the correct or 'healthy' frequency, and entraining the oscillations back to coherence.

These are profoundly significant concepts for all therapeutic approaches to the body. The whole field of chemical analysis by spectroscopy shows that there is a 'fundamental duality between chemical structure and coherent oscillations'. Coherent vibrations in living systems are as fundamental as chemical bonds (Smith 1994). There are two ways of altering functions in the body: one is to add particular molecules to the system, and the other is to add the electromagnetic signature of those molecules. The energy fields projected from the hands of bodyworkers are in the range of intensity and frequency that can influence regulatory processes within the body of another person.

Energy fields can have profound biological and psychological effects, particularly if they are applied at or near certain active regions on the skin (Andreev et al 1984). Many studies have demonstrated interactions between cells and molecules that are not touching (reviewed by Smith 1994). The most intriguing and clinically significant examples come from research on homeopathy and related vibrational medicines, which we shall consider in the next chapter.

References

Adolph E F 1979 Look at physiological integration. American Journal of Physiology 237:R255–R259

Adolph E F 1982 Physiological integrations in action. Physiologist 25:Supplement 2

Allen H C, Cross P C 1963 Molecular Vib-rotors. John Wiley, New York

Andreev E A, Beloy M V, Sitko S P 1984 The manifestation of natural characteristic frequencies of the organism of man. Reports to the Academy of Sciences of the Ukrainian SSR No. 10, Series b, Geological, Chemical and Biological Sciences, pp 60–63

Athenstaedt H 1974 Pyroelectric and piezoelectric properties of vertebrates. Annals of the New York Academy of Sciences 238:68–94

Ball K 1994 Designing the molecular world: chemistry at the frontier. Princeton University Press, Princeton, NJ

Barrett S, Jarvis W T 1993 The health robbers: a close look at quackery in America. Prometheus Books, Buffalo, NY

Bouligand Y 1978 Liquid crystals and their analogs in biological systems. In: Liebert L (ed) Liquid crystals. Solid State Physics, Supplement 14:259–294

Callahan P S 1975 Tuning into nature. Devin-Adair, Greenwich, CT

Crim F F 1990 State- and bond-selected unimolecular reactions. Science 249:1387

Del Giudice E, Preparata G, Vitiello G 1988 Water as a free electric dipole laser. Physical Review Letters 61:1085–1088

Fröhlich H 1975 The extraordinary dielectric properties of biological molecules and the action of enzymes. Proceedings of the National Academy of Sciences of the USA 72:4211–4215

Fröhlich H 1978 Coherent electric vibrations in biological systems and the cancer problem. IEEE Transactions on Microwave Theory and Techniques MTT 26:613–617

Galde P 1991 Crystal healing. Llewellyn Publications, St Paul, MN

Gerber R 1988 Vibrational medicine. Bear, Santa Fe, NM

Gilson M K, Straatsma T P, McCammon J A et al 1994 Open 'back door' in a molecular dynamics simulation of acetylcholinesterase. Science 263:1276–1278

Goodsell D S 1993 The machinery of life. Springer-Verlag, New York

Grundler W, Keilmann F, Fröhlich H 1977 Resonant growth rate response of yeast cells irradiated by weak microwaves. Physics Letters 62A:463–466

Ho M-W 1993 The rainbow and the worm: the physics of organisms. World Scientific, River Edge, NJ

Jeffery K 1993 Seashells as massage tools. Massage Therapy Journal (Spring):72–73

Karplus M, McCammon J A 1986 The dynamics of proteins: the incessant motions that underlie a protein's function are explored in computer simulations. Scientific American 254:42–51

Mellor D J 1966 A physiological integration. Drug Houses of Australia Ltd, Medical Division, PO Box 4746, Melbourne, Vic 3000, Australia

Pauling L 1960 The nature of the chemical bond and the structure of molecules and crystals, 3rd edn. Cornell University Press, Ithaca, NY

Popp F A, Ruth B, Bahr W et al 1981 Emission of visible and ultraviolet radiation by active biological systems. Collective Phenomena 3:187–214

Popp F A, Li K H, Gu Q 1992 Recent advances in biophoton research. World Scientific, Singapore

Preparata G 1995 QED coherence in matter. World Scientific, River Edge, NJ

Rasmussen H 1981 Calcium and cAMP as synarchic messengers. John Wiley & Sons, New York

Raso J 1995 Mystical medical alternativism. Skeptical Inquirer 19(5):33–37

Sauer K (ed) 1995 Biochemical spectroscopy. Methods in Enzymology 246. Academic Press, New York

Smith C W 1994 Biological effects of weak electromagnetic fields. In: Ho M W, Popp F-A, Warnke U (eds) Bioelectrodynamics and biocommunication. World Scientific, Singapore, ch 3, pp 81–107

Szent-Györgyi A 1963 Lost in the twentieth century. Annual Review of Biochemistry 32:1–14

Weisskopf V F 1968 How light interacts with matter: the everyday objects around us are white, colored or black, opaque or transparent, depending on how the electrons in their atoms or molecules respond to the driving force of electromagnetic radiation. Scientific American 219:60–71

Whiffen D H 1966 Spectroscopy. John Wiley and Sons, Chichester, p 102

10 Homeopathy and related vibrational medicines

What is urgently needed is to be able to read the language of
electromagnetic biocommunication to complement our understanding of
the genetic code.
C.W. Smith (1994)

Rationale for vibrational medicines

The rationale behind vibrational medicine is straightforward: diseases and disorders alter the electromagnetic properties of molecules, cells, tissues, and organs. In addition to the familiar regulatory systems studied by physiologists, the human body contains an electromagnetic control network. Ancient methods such as acupuncture recognize, understand and treat via these systems. Modern research is determining their biophysical mechanisms and electromagnetic 'languages'.

When a particular molecule is deficient or altered or in excess because of a disease or disorder, normal functioning can sometimes be restored with a drug. This is the basis for pharmacology. Vibrational medicines such as homeopathy demonstrate that similar or even better results can be obtained by providing the electromagnetic fingerprint or signature of a natural substance (Smith 1994). In the previous chapter, we coined the term 'energetic pharmacology' to distinguish this approach from conventional chemical pharmacology.

A substance, or its electromagnetic signature, challenges the defense and repair systems to respond, without the side-effects of pharmacological interventions. In some cases an imbalanced system is restored by introducing a signal that cancels a discordant or pathological frequency that is disturbing the body.

In bodywork and movement therapies, the emanations from a therapist's own tissues can provide electromagnetic information that opens or augments vital communications in a patient's tissues. Light and sound therapists apply energies of particular frequencies to appropriate points on the body (e.g. 'colorpuncture', Mandel 1986).

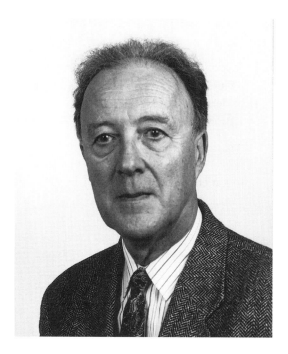

Fig. 10.1 Dr Cyril W. Smith. (Portrait used with permission from Dr Cyril W. Smith. Photograph by Invicta Studio, Manchester.)

These energetic approaches are not based on vague or obscure theories. For example, studies of energetic phenomena have provided most of the images of atoms and molecules shown in chemistry and biochemistry texts. Spectroscopy is the general field of study, and a series of Nobel prizes attest to its significance. Developments in spectroscopy are closely linked to quantum theory and to our understanding of the fundamental nature of all matter, both animate and inanimate. Astronomers and astrophysicists use spectroscopic methods to determine the composition of stars and other objects that are too far away to allow close-up study.

Medical spectroscopy and the 'water system'

Biomedical scientists are beginning to use spectroscopic methods in the detection and cure of diseases (Jackson & Mantsch 1996). Their results confirm what energy therapists have known for a long time: the human body emits vibratory information that precisely specifies the activities taking place within. We saw in Chapter 1 that Harold Saxton Burr reached a similar conclusion, many years ago.

Modern researchers are generally unaware of the extensive background exploration done by the founders of various vibrational medicines, and by those who have carefully and thoughtfully continued these lines of inquiry.

Magnetic resonance imaging (MRI) is a spectroscopic method that is widely and successfully used for medical diagnosis. MRI works because tumours contain abnormal arrangements of water (Damadian 1971, Damadian et al 1974). Most physiologists attach no significance to this important fact, as they do not recognize that the body has a 'water system' involved in communication and regulation. As with the electrocardiogram, medical science accepts the information provided by MRI images as a sort of by-product of life, without appreciating the profoundly important energy picture that underlies the method. In contrast, homeopathy and other vibrational medicines take advantage of the water system and its great sensitivity to electromagnetic fields.

Living tissues contain thousands of different kinds of molecules, each of which is surrounded by water (Watterson 1988). Until recently, the medical use of direct body spectroscopy has been hampered by the fact that cell and tissue water absorbs the radiations one would like to study. The scientific question is what the water molecules 'do' with the absorbed information. Do they convert it to random processes (heat)? Or do the water molecules do something more sophisticated? Can water molecules store molecular signatures? Can such information be conducted through the water system? Perhaps the troubling 'artifact' of water absorption actually explains how homeopathic dilutions and the body's water system absorb information from a substance.

While the subject continues to be highly controversial, a number of scientists have reversed their opinions from insisting that the phenomenon of 'water memory' is impossible, to determining the mechanisms involved. A key step was the publication in 1994 of a scholarly book entitled *Ultra High Dilution Physiology and Physics* (Endler & Schulte 1994). Scientists from 10 countries contributed essays to the collection. Current thinking is that 'water memory' does not violate any laws of physics or nature. It simply means that our understanding of water is incomplete.

In homeopathy, molecular signatures are transferred from a biologically active molecule to the water in which it is dissolved. This happens when the homeopathic physician 'succusses' the sample. Succussion is a method of vibrating or sending a shock wave through a solution. Dissolved molecules are made to vibrate intensely and coherently, and they therefore emit their electromagnetic signatures (emission spectrum).

One plausible mechanism for water memory storage, published by Smith (1985), is that hydrogen bonds hold water molecules together in a helical structure that acts like a coil. The magnetic components of fields emitted by the vibrating molecules induce current flows through the water helix. These currents reverberate within the water structure, much like the ringing of a tuning fork.

Even when the sample has been diluted to the point that the original molecule is gone, the signals stored in the water continue to vibrate for a long time. Upon further dilution and succussion, the reverberating signals transfer to other water molecules used to dilute the sample.

The ability of atomic systems to recall coherent electromagnetic pulses is known to physicists (Brewer & Hahn 1984). Several independent reports document storage of information by water (e.g. Trincher 1980).

Studies of allergic reactions

C. W. Smith (Fig. 10.1) has developed important clinical applications of vibrational medicine (Smith 1988, 1994). His results are important to those who suffer from a wide range of ailments.

The significance of Smith's studies for bodywork and movement therapists is that they document the astonishing sensitivity of physiological regulatory systems to electromagnetic fields. Moreover, every therapist has a few clients with frustrating conditions that do not respond to treatment. The patient may have an electromagnetic allergy, a condition rarely recognized by medicine. Those who are hypersensitive to 60-cycle electricity may develop dizziness, nausea or migraines that are triggered by walking past a hidden transformer or by standing next to an appliance such as a toaster. Sometimes physicians give drugs to treat the symptoms, the drugs produce side-effects, and more drugs are given to treat those side-effects. Some of these individuals will benefit immediately by being made aware of how their electromagnetic environment is affecting them (see Becker 1990). The best way of checking one's environment for strong magnetic fields is to use a simple detector (see Chapter 14 and Appendix I).

Since 1982, Smith has studied more than 100 electrically sensitive multiple-allergy patients. Smith explains how regulatory systems (such as shown in

Fig. 9.8) can be set into chaos by minute quantities of chemicals or by energy fields in the environment. Just as harmful chemicals can disrupt body chemistry and cause disease, harmful electromagnetic fields can sensitize and disrupt electronic signaling within the organism.

Multiple allergic responses are acquired when a patient is exposed to a previously innocuous substance or frequency while reacting to an allergen. In extreme cases, an individual may react to as many as 100 different stimuli.

Allergic reactions can be triggered by specific electromagnetic frequencies in the range of a few thousandths of a hertz to a gigahertz (one billion cycles per second). Moreover, Smith found that other electromagnetic fields, of appropriate frequencies, can halt the reaction. According to Smith, 'the pattern of allergic responses is the same whether the trigger is chemical, environmental, nutritional or electrical' (Smith 1988).

Traditional therapy for allergies has involved pricking the skin with a diluted allergen. The result is a weal on the skin. As the allergen is taken through a series of dilutions, the weal gets smaller, then larger, then smaller, etc., until a dilution is reached where no weal is produced. This is known as the patient's 'neutralizing dilution' and can be injected to protect the patient from subsequent exposure – a sort of immunization.

Work by Monro and colleagues (cited in Smith 1988) showed that extremely sensitive allergy patients needed only to hold a glass tube containing a dilution of the allergen to show symptoms or neutralizing effects. The most sensitive patients could even distinguish tubes of allergen that were merely brought into the same room.

Smith and his colleagues used electromagnetic fields from an adjustable oscillator to test and treat electrically hypersensitive allergy patients. Increasing the frequency has the same effect as diluting the allergen. Eventually a frequency is reached that has the same effect as the 'neutralizing dilution'.

The studies are begun with the signal generator in the adjacent room to see if the patient can tell whether the signals are on or off. For sensitive patients, the signal generator does not even need to have an antenna attached to its output terminals. For less sensitive patients, a short length of wire is adequate. In no case is the wire physically connected to the patient. The amounts of radiation are no larger than that leaking from a television set or home computer.

Lakhovsky used high frequency fields to treat cancer. His theory (Lakhovsky 1939) was that health involved a balance or equilibrium in the electrical oscillations in living cells, and that disease arises from oscillatory disequilibrium.

While medical science dismissed Lakhovsky's approach for over 50 years, his theory coincides with the concepts that are now emerging from the work of Fröhlich, Smith, Bassett, Endler, Schulte, and others discussed in this book. Acupuncture, electroacupuncture, colourpuncture, and a variety of other 'energy therapies' are also based on balancing energy systems in the body.

The frequency range 1–30 Hz is particularly important physiologically and is also the frequency of normal variations in the geomagnetic field. Of particular interest are the ELF frequencies present in all human subjects and that resonate with homeopathic remedies. Ludwig (1987) has reported on the resonant frequencies of particular physiological functions in man.

Studies on bacteria and yeasts indicate that specific coherent frequencies can trigger proliferation. This may be a part of the Candida problem. For example, the clocks in computers operate at frequencies that can be biologically active. One of Smith's allergy patients had attacks of colitis that seemed to be triggered by working next to a computer with an 8 MHz (8 million cycles per second) clock frequency. This frequency affects the growth of yeasts (Aarholt et al 1981).

Not only can patients be extremely sensitive to electromagnetic fields, they can also emit signals during their allergic reactions. These signals can actually be large enough to produce allergic reactions in sensitive individuals nearby.

Electronic devices have been developed to detect signals from allergic patients, phase invert them, and feed them back into the body for therapeutic purposes. These methods are based on connecting a sophisticated electronic circuit to particular acupuncture meridians related to specific organ systems (Gerber 1988, Scott-Mumby 1999). Some of these instruments can perform hundreds of tests for allergic responses in a few seconds, using a frequency-matching system. The body is checked for responses to molecular signatures that have been digitized and stored in a computer.

While a 'personal oscillator' set to a patient's neutralizing frequency might seem to be an effective treatment for an allergy, the correct frequency for one person can be another's allergic trigger. Because of this, a better method is to expose a vial of mineral water to the patient's neutralizing frequency. The patient can merely hold the vial of water in his or her hand to neutralize an allergic reaction. The water retains its effectiveness for at least 1–2 months. However, if the patient undergoes a strong allergic reaction, the water seems to lose its effectiveness. Smith thinks this happens because such patients emit signals that 'overwrite' the signal stored in the water.

We have presented a few of the fascinating and important discoveries and clinical applications of vibrational medicine. Those who have had satisfactory clinical outcomes tend to be disinterested in the scientific debates, and are instead simply grateful that they feel better.

Some conclusions

Much of the seeming magic and mystery surrounding vibrational medicines is being revealed as the same mystery, that has always been associated with the invisible yet palpable forces of nature. Many of the subtleties arising in the clinical context are none other than the subtleties of human structure and patterns of energy in interaction. As new research reveals the basis for these subtleties, we obtain a much clearer picture of the human body in health and disease. The medical and chemical-pharmacological models that have served us well in the past are not being replaced, but are being viewed within a more complete multidimensional perspective. 'Subtle energies' and 'dynamic energy systems' are neither supernatural nor do they require a revision of physics. They go to the foundation of life. The molecules and energy fields in our environment can affect living systems. An understanding of these relationships, whether based on intuition or on science, is fundamental to a wide range of therapeutic approaches, including flower essences, homeopathy, aromatherapy, sound and light therapy, the use of crystals, and many others.

References

Aarholt E, Flinn EA, Smith CW 1981 Effects of low frequency magnetic fields on bacterial growth rate. Physics in Medicine and Biology 76: 613–621

Becker RO 1990 Cross Currents: the promise of electromedicine, the perils of electropollution. Jeremy P Tarcher, Los Angeles, CA

Brewer RH, Hahn EL 1984 Atomic memory. Scientific American 241: 50–57

Damadian R 1971 Tumor detection by nuclear magnetic resonance. Science 171: 1151–1153

Damadian R, Zner K, Hor D, DiMaio T 1974 Human tumors detected by nuclear magnetic resonance. Proceedings of the National Academy of Sciences of the USA 71: 1471–1473

Endler PC, Schulte J 1994 Ultra high dilution physiology and physics. Kluwer Academic, Dordrecht

Gerber R 1988 Vibrational medicine Bear, Santa Fe, NM, pp. 221–222

Jackson M, Mantsch HH 1996 Biomedical infrared spectroscopy. In: Mantsch HH, Chapman D (eds) Infrared spectroscopy of biomolecules. Wiley-Liss, New York, pp. 311–340

Lakhovsky G 1939 The secret of life. Heinemann Medical, London

Ludwig HW 1987 Electromagnetic multiresonance – the base of homeopathy and biophysical therapy. In: Proceedings of the 42nd Congress of the International Homeopathic Medical League, 29 March–2 April 1987, Arlington, American Institute of Homeopathy, Washington, DC

Mandel P 1986 Colorpuncture. Energetik Verlag, Bruchsal, Germany

Scott-Mumby K 1999 Virtual medicine. Thorsons/Harper Collins, London

Smith CW 1985 Superconducting areas in living systems. In: Mishra RK (ed) The Living State II. World Scientific, Singapore, pp. 404–420

Smith CW 1988 Electromagnetic effects in humans. In: Fröhlich H (ed) Biological coherence and response to external stimuli. Springer-Verlag, Berlin, pp. 205–232

Smith CW 1994 Biological effects of weak electromagnetic fields. In: Ho M-W, Popp F-A, Warnke U (eds) Bioelectrodynamics and biocommunication. World Scientific, Singapore, pp. 81–107

Trincher K 1980 The information content of intracellular water and its accumulation in embryo- and phyloogenesis. Biological Cybernetics 39: 1–10

Watterson JG 1988 The role of water in cell architecture. Molecular and Cellular Biochemistry 79: 101–105

11 Gravity, structure, emotions

Introduction

Previous chapters have described the physiological and clinical importance of electricity and magnetism. Little has been said about gravity, even though it is arguably the most potent physical influence in any human life.

Gravity pervades our bodies and our environment and affects our every activity. All of the structures around us – our homes, furniture, buildings, machinery, plants and animals – and our own bodies, are designed to function in a world dominated by gravity. The form of each bone, muscle, and sinew tells a story of its particular role in maintaining and moving the body in the gravitational field. Many of the injuries faced in the therapeutic setting are consequences of falling down, or of habitual movement patterns that strain tissues. Hence therapists of virtually every tradition can benefit from an appreciation of the ways in which gravity interacts with structures, energy flows, and emotions, and the clinical approaches that remedy 'gravitational traumas'.

Gravitational physiology

To introduce the therapeutic significance of gravity, we summarize the work of Joel E. Goldthwait and his colleagues at Harvard Medical School. Their clinical research in the early part of the 20th century laid an important but rarely cited foundation for modern bodywork and movement therapies.

A surgeon in Boston and founder of the orthopaedic clinic at the Massachusetts General Hospital, Goldthwait developed a successful therapeutic approach to chronic disorders. The aim of his therapies was to get his patients to sit, stand, and move with their bodies in a more appropriate relationship with the vertical. After years of treating patients with chronic problems, he concluded that many of these problems arise because parts of the body become misaligned with respect to the vertical, and organ functions therefore become compromised.

Goldthwait's therapeutic approach was based in part on observations made while performing surgery on such patients. He noticed that abdominal nerves and blood vessels are under tension in individuals whose bodies are out of alignment. He also reported 'stretching and kinking' of the cerebral arteries and veins in those whose necks were bent. Various cardiac problems were correlated with 'faulty body mechanics' that distorted the chest cavity in a way that impaired circulatory efficiency. Goldthwait also documented with X-rays a build-up of calcium deposits around the vertebrae of individuals with chronic arthritis, and observed that these deposits can diminish when the individual acquires a more vertical stance (Fig. 11.1). His therapeutic approach corrected many difficult problems without the use of drugs. He viewed the human body from a mechanical engineering perspective, in which alignment of parts is essential to reduce wear and stress. He pleaded with physicians to recognize and correct misalignments to prevent long-term harmful effects.

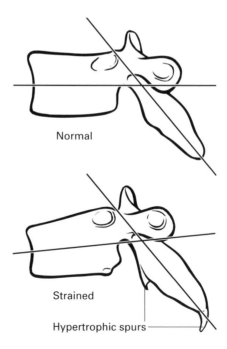

Normal

Strained

Hypertrophic spurs

Fig. 11.1 Goldthwait's drawings of a normal vertebra and one showing the effects of longstanding strain and pressure from 'faulty body mechanics' as occurs in a rounded or drooped dorsal spine. The strained vertebra shows: narrowing of the anterior region; the spinous process is at a more acute angle from the vertebral body; the arch of the intervertebral foremen is narrower; evidences of strain include the hypertrophic spurs on the articular facets and the tip of the spinous process. (After Goldthwait et al 1934, Fig. 10, p. 25.)

Goldthwait's observations and concepts, and those of others in the field (e.g. Strait et al 1947, Hellebrandt & Franseen 1943) are important and fascinating. However, research of this kind was begun at the dawn of the era of pharmacology. Medical inquiry was soon swept away in the tide of drug-based medicine that continues today.

In articles published in 1909 and 1911, Goldthwait wrote an impassioned plea for everyone to pay more attention to the ways they hold and move their bodies in relation to the gravity field. While Goldthwait's concepts did not become established in clinical medicine, a number of modern schools of bodywork and movement therapies rely on similar principles:

> The way we hold and move our bodies in our daily activities is more important than most people realize. It is desirable to be able to stand erect and to have the parts of the body balanced so that easy and graceful movement occur. These ideas about how we stand and move are important for full health and economic efficiency of the body. The most economical way to use the body is with proper poise. This allows more energy to be available for whatever task is required. Any time a structure departs from the balanced state, energy is wasted and efficiency is reduced. An imbalance can cause one part of the body to be strained more than another, but no one part can be strained without affecting the whole body.

> It would seem to be a matter simply of common sense to expect better health with the body so poised or balanced that all of the organs are in their proper positions and the muscles are in proper balance. Likewise with the poise such that the viscera of both the abdomen and thorax must be out of place, as can easily be demonstrated with X-rays, the best health could hardly be expected. The malposition of an organ will disturb its function. If malposition continues long enough, permanent damage will result, but if the faulty mechanics is corrected, damage will be prevented.

Goldthwait and his colleagues (1934) identified several 'grades' of body mechanics (Fig. 11.2). Texts on biomechanics and Rolfing® (Rolf 1977) analyze the relation of the body with the vertical by imagining a plumb bob attached to a point at the centre of the head and dropped through the body structure (Fig. 11.2E). In the illustration, we have defined Rolf's 'gravity line' and superimposed it on Goldthwait's drawings. The experienced bodyworker will notice that the body shown in Figure 11.2A, which Goldthwait identifies as 'excellent mechanical use of the body', still exhibits strain and departure from verticality.

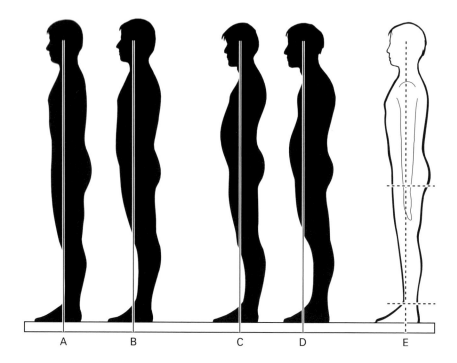

Fig. 11.2 **A–D** are from The Harvard University Chart for Grading Body Mechanics (Goldthwait et al 1934). The images are described as follows: **A** Excellent mechanical use of the body. Head straight above chest. hips and feet; chest up and forward, abdomen in or flat, back, usual curves not exaggerated. **B** Good mechanical use of the body. Head too far forward; chest not so well up or forward; abdomen and back, very little change. **C** Poor mechanical use of the body. Head forward of chest; chest flat; abdomen relaxed and forward; back curves are exaggerated. **D** very poor mechanical use of the body. Head still farther forward; chest still flatter and farther back; abdomen completely relaxed, 'slouchy' back, all curves exaggerated to the extreme. (A–D from Goldthwait et al 1934, p. 8, with permission from Arnold.) **E** The ideal vertical structure defined by Ida P. Rolf in her classic book on Rolfing® (Rolf 1977). The ideal 'gravity line' passes through the ear (bisecting the external meatus), the shoulder (head of the humerus), hip bone (head of the femur), knee and ankle (external malleolus). (After Rolf 1977) Figure redrawn with permission from JB Lippincott, Alan Demmerle, John Lodge and the Rolf Institute.)

A legacy of the Victorian era is a belief that better poise is the result of better posture. Children are still admonished to sit, stand and walk in a more erect manner. We now know that there is much more to the story. Modern body-workers and movement therapists are aware that accumulated trauma can gradually cause the body to depart from alignment with the vertical. For many individuals, such as those shown in Figure 11.2 B–D, it is simply impossible to force their bodies into an upright posture. Injuries, traumas, habitual movement patterns, or prolonged sitting in poorly designed furniture gradually alter body structure in ways that compromise verticality and that affect well-being. For these individuals, no amount of admonishing them to 'stand up straight' can enable them to assume a vertical stance.

To understand how the body can gradually depart from verticality, how this influences health and energetic efficiency, and how verticality can be restored, we need to explore the 'gravity system' of the body.

A gravity system

The muscles, their connective tissue or fascial coverings, and their connections to the tendons, bones, ligaments, and cartilages, support us in the gravity field and enable us to move and act upon our environment. The 'gravity system' of the body consists of the motor nerves, muscles, connective tissues, and sensory systems that monitor the motion, tension, and position of every part, and provide our kinesthetic experience.

In describing the ways the body responds to injury and to clinical procedures, it is useful to look at the relations between the various connective tissue systems. All of the great systems of the body – the skin, nervous system, musculature, digestive tract, circulatory system, lymphatics, skeleton, and the various organs – have their characteristic forms and properties because of the connective tissues they are composed of. In other words, connective tissue is a ubiquitous and versatile biological material that forms and interconnects all of the components of the living body.

Simple mechanical calculations reveal that gravity gives rise to surprisingly large forces within the body. The reason for this is that the musculoskeletal system has a number of simple levers that amplify the forces exerted on joints and other tissues (Fig. 11.3).

The tensegrity concept is a useful way to conceptualize the interconnected gravitational support/energetic system in the body.

Tensegrity

Tensegrity is an architectural principle developed in 1948 by R. Buckminster Fuller. The tensegrity principle underlies geodesic domes, tents, sailing vessels,

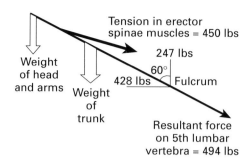

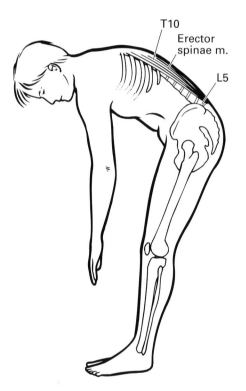

Fig. 11.3 Forces arising in the lower back region during bending. The calculations are based on a simple model of a man weighing 180 lb. The fifth lumbar vertebra is regarded as the fulcrum for the spine, and the erector spinae muscles are considered cables. Equilibrium is achieved when muscular forces balance the pull of gravity plus the weight of a load being lifted. Without lifting a weight, the compressive force on the 5th lumbar vertebra is 494 lb. Should the man be lifting a 50-lb load in the position shown, the compressive force on the 5th lumbar increases to 855 lb. (Illustrations and calculations are from Strait et al 1947, Fig. 5, p. 377, and Fig. 6, p. 378 with permission from the American Journal of Physiology and the American Physiological Society.)

and various stick-and-wire sculptures and toy models (Pugh 1976). A tensegrity system is characterized by a continuous tensional network (tendons) connected by a discontinuous set of compressive elements (struts). A tensegrity structure forms a stable yet dynamic system that interacts efficiently and resiliently with forces acting upon it (Fig. 11.4).

Tensegrity provides a conceptual link between the structural systems and the energy/informational systems we have been discussing in this book. The body as a whole, and the spine in particular, can usefully be described as tensegrity systems (Robbie 1977). In the body, bones act as discontinuous compression elements and the muscles, tendons and ligaments act as a continuous tensional system. Together the bones and tensional elements permit the body to change shape, move about and lift objects. Robbie (1977) reaches the remarkable conclusion that the soft tissues around the spine, when under appropriate tension, can actually lift each vertebra off the one below it. He views the spine as a tensegrity mast.

The various ligaments form 'slings' that are capable of supporting the weight of the body without applying compressive forces to the vertebrae and intervertebral discs. In other words, the vertebral column is not, as it is usually portrayed, a simple stack of blocks, each cushioned by an intervertebral disc. The basis for this concept is illustrated and summarized in Figure 11.5.

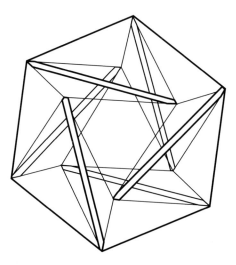

Fig. 11.4 A simple tensegrity system. Tensegrity structures contain a continuous system of tendons and a discontinuous set of compression members called struts.

The tensegrity system of a rabbit is shown in Figure 11.6. This remarkable diagram from a book by Young (1957) was obtained by representing each muscle–tendon combination as a single straight line. Figure 11.7 shows how the tensegrity concept applies equally to a bone and to a lifting device such as a crane.

When applied to the myofascial system, the tensegrity concept explains the ability of the body to absorb impacts without being damaged. Mechanical energy flows away from a site of impact as an elastic shock wave in the tensegrous network. The more flexible and balanced and communicative the network, the more readily it absorbs shocks. This is important in understand-

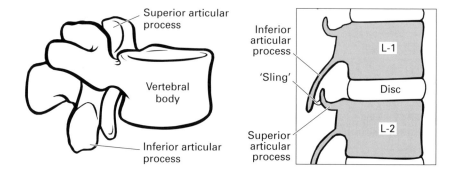

Fig. 11.5 Robbie (1977) has concluded that the soft tissues around the spine, when under appropriate tension, can actually lift each vertebra off the one below it. Robbie notes that the vertebral bodies contain little of the compact bone or trabeculae commonly associated with weight-bearing bones of the body. Instead, the lumbar vertebrae, which supposedly support the weight of the body plus any additional loads being carried by the person, are composed mainly of cancellous or spongy bone. The parts of the vertebra that seem well designed for weight-bearing are the paired articular processes, which are composed of thick layers of compact bone. The upward projecting superior articular processes of one vertebra are situated higher than the lower tips of the downward projecting inferior articular process of the vertebra above it. The fibrous connective tissue connecting these processes forms 'slings' that suspend each vertebra from the one below it. Hence the spine can be viewed both as a stack of blocks and as a tensegrity mast. People with back disorders involving compressed or herniated intervertebral discs may have spines that are functioning primarily in the 'stack of blocks' mode. Therapies that strengthen or tone the ligaments and myofascias associated with the spine can shift the spine into a more tensegrous mode, and thereby relieve the pressure on the discs. To the left is a drawing of a lumbar vertebra (after Warwick & Williams 1973, Fig. 3.39, p. 240, with permission). (The drawing to the right is after Robbie 1977, Fig. 1, p. 46. Tensional forces in the human body. Orthopaedic Review VI(11), November issue, p. 46 with permission from the publisher copyright © 1977 by Quadrant Healthcom Inc.)

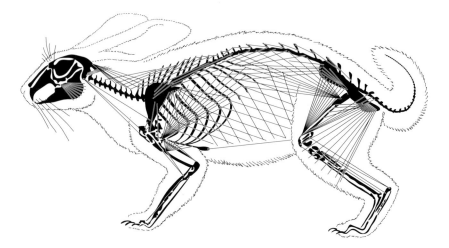

Fig. 11.6 A drawing of a tensegrity system of a rabbit, created by replacing each muscle–tendon unit with a single straight line. (Reproduced from a figure drawn from life or redrawn from another figure by Miss ER Turlington and Miss JID de Vere in Young Z 1957 The Life of Mammals. Oxford University Press, New York, with kind permission from Oxford University Press.)

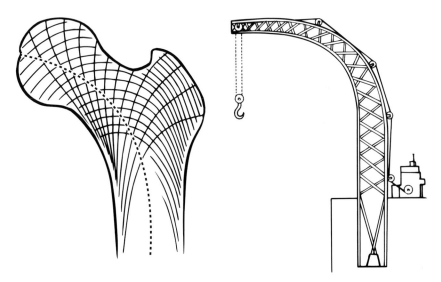

Fig. 11.7 The head of the femur and a crane are both tensegrity structures, as they employ both compression and tension resisting elements.

ing how flexible and organized fascial continuities can reduce the incidence of injury to athletes and other performers.

As Goldthwait stated in 1909, an imbalance can cause one part of the body to be strained more than another, but no one part can be strained without affecting the whole body. Inflexibility or shortening in one tissue influences structure and movement in other parts. The 'anatomy trains' documented by Myers (1997a, 1997b) explain how local injuries can influence distant tissues, and even create a predisposition for new injuries.

Just as a strain in one area of the body affects the whole body, an improvement in flexibility in one area will have effects that radiate outward, particularly along the fascial 'trains' mentioned above. While a therapist may focus attention on a particular region that is stiff or inflexible or painful, beneficial effects can, and do, spread to other areas. Moreover, the modern bodyworker is aware that problems in areas that are too painful to be touched can nonetheless benefit from work done on nearby areas. The success of such approaches is due to tensional continuity, and to the fact that the living tensegrity system is a continuous semiconductor vibratory network. This can be demonstrated with a tensegrity model by plucking one of the tendons, which causes the entire network to vibrate.

In hands-on bodywork, and particularly in energetic bodywork, the vibrations consist of the oscillating energy fields emitted from the hands. These vibrations, in turn, consist of a blend of the fields generated by molecular, cellular, tissue, and systemic oscillations within the body of the therapist. In other therapeutic approaches, other forms of energy – such as laser light, sound, electric, or magnetic fields, or heat are applied to particular points on the surface of the body. The semiconducting tensegrous network absorbs these energies and converts them into acoustic vibrations of various frequencies (Hyman et al 1981, Saleh & Teich 1991, Oschman 1993) that propagate throughout the system.

Since the tensegrity network is simultaneously a mechanical and a vibratory continuum, restrictions in one part have both structural and energetic consequences for the entire organism. Structural integrity and vibratory, or energetic, or informational integrity go hand in hand – one cannot influence the structural system without influencing the energetic/informational system, and vice versa.

Tensegrity on the cellular scale

Cells and nuclei are tensegrity systems (Coffey 1985, Ingber & Jamieson 1985, Ingber & Folkman 1989). Elegant research has documented how the gravity system connects, via a family of molecules known as integrins, to the cytoskeletons of cells throughout the body. Integrins 'glue' every cell in the body to neighbouring cells and to the surrounding connective tissue matrix. An important study by Wang et al (1993) documents that integrin molecules carry tension from the extracellular matrix, across the cell surface, to the cytoskeleton, which behaves as a tensegrity matrix. Ingber (1993a, 1993b) has shown how cell shape and function are regulated by an interacting tension and compression system within the cytoskeleton (see Ch. 4 and Figs 4.3 and 4.6).

A recent article by Horwitz (1997) documents the increasing awareness among medical researchers that integrins regulate most functions of the body and play key roles in arthritis, heart disease, stroke, osteoporosis, and the spread of cancer. Research on integrins and their attachments has profound significance for movement therapy and bodywork. The reason is that integrin molecules are focal points where many approaches converge, in terms of physiology, biochemistry, energetics, emotions, and therapeutic technique. Of particular interest are the roles of the integrins in the migrations of cells that defend the body against disease and repair injuries (Lauffenburger & Horwitz 1996, Hynes 1992).

Plasticity

Physical structure and movement patterns are plastic – they can adapt to the ways the body is used. Plasticity of the nervous system is demonstrated by abrupt changes in movement patterns in response to injury. For example, a sprained ankle immediately leads to a limp – a temporary movement pattern that takes pressure off the injured part until it heals. Plasticity of both bones and soft tissues is demonstrated by the laying down of collagen fibers in tissues that are called upon to carry extra weight, and by the removal of excess collagen when loading is reduced. The mechanism was described over a century ago By Wolff: 'The form of the bone (or other connective tissue) being given, the bone elements (collagen) place or displace themselves in the direction of the functional pressure and increase or decrease their mass to reflect the amount of functional pressure.' (Wolff 1892)

The mechanisms by which cells lay down or resorb supporting materials (collagen) in bone and connective tissue are understood. Electric fields generated during movements (Fig. 3.5) signal cells (fibroblasts in connective tissue, osteoblasts in bone) to lay down collagen in the direction of tension, and thereby strengthen the tissues. With less loading or movement, the electric fields are weaker and less frequent, and the cells resorb collagen (Bassett 1968).

Related processes are involved in wound healing, and are well documented. For example, Weiss (1961) found that wound repair begins with formation of a clot containing randomly oriented fibers (Fig. 11.8). As the clot dissolves, fibers not under tension dissolve first, leaving only fibers oriented along the lines of tension. Fibroblast cells migrate into the web and become oriented along the tension fibers. Where the damage is to the support system of the body, the energetic sequence involves gravity, which introduces tension (elastic energy) to the tissue, which generates electricity (piezoelectric effect and streaming potentials), which signals cells to migrate (by cytoskeletal 'motors' that consume chemical energy), and the cells then lay down collagen.

The biochemical basis for tissue plasticity or remodeling was worked out over 50 years ago, when Rudolph Schoenheimer MD of Columbia University reported his pioneering studies in which radioactive isotopes were used to label organic compounds that could be included in the diets of animals. The labeled molecules could be traced to see if they became incorporated into the tissues of the animal, or were excreted.

Biologists had considered the structure of the adult body to be relatively fixed and permanent, although a few had suggested that a small portion of the dietary intake might be used to repair and replace structures that undergo wear and tear. Schoenheimer and his colleagues discovered that a large fraction of

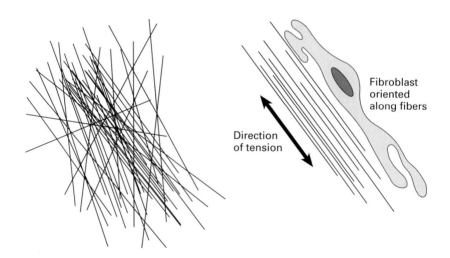

Fig. 11.8 Weiss (1961) found that wound repair begins with formation of a clot containing randomly oriented fibers. As the clot dissolves, fibers not under tension dissolve first, leaving only fibers oriented along the lines of tension. Fibroblast cells migrate into the web and become oriented along the tension fibers. Fibroblasts lay down collagen along lines of tension.

the tagged compounds in the diet were rapidly incorporated into tissues. On the basis of these findings, Schoenheimer (1942) developed a concept of 'metabolic regeneration' that has stood the test of time (Ratner 1979). Components of the body are constantly being assembled and disassembled. The rates of assembly and disassembly are normally in balance, so that body parts remain nearly constant in quantity, position, and structure. The lytic or degradative enzymes that take structures apart are balanced by synthetic or generative reactions. These enzymes are proteins that are also constantly being assembled and taken apart. The process is controlled by the cell nucleus, which fine-tunes the rates of production and degradation of the enzymes. Each tissue in the body has a different rate of turnover.

Metabolic regeneration allows for rapid adaptation of an organism's structure in response to changes in movement patterns. Schonheimer's research explains how practice can gradually allow the bodies of athletes, musicians, dancers, and other performers to adapt in structure, function, and motion. An extreme example is the bodybuilder, who through the stimulus of constant exertion, brings about a dramatic alteration in body form. Not only do the muscles increase in size and strength, but other components of the myofascial system increase as well. The delicate skill of the concert violinist is an example of the same phenomenon – the gradual perfection of form and motion as the body strives to adapt or 'optimize itself' to the ways it is used. In all of these examples, there is a coordinated change in all of the structures and functions involved. Likewise, various kinds of bodywork and movement therapy can change patterns of movement, and thereby change patterns of electrical fields that arise from that movement, and this ultimately leads to changes in body structure.

Pickup (1978) described how behaviorally-mediated patterns of stress can bring about increases in collagen density. Young (1957) pointed out that the pattern of collagen fibers represents a sort of 'memory' of the ways the body has been used or abused. Bodyworkers and movement therapists sense the restrictions to structure or movement patterns caused by dense tissue. We have described recent research showing that Young's concept also applies to the cellular parts of the tensegrity network (Oschman & Oschman 1994a, 1994b). A holographic model of memory is consistent with the 'somatic recall' phenomenon, in which application of pressure to a particular area releases a vivid recollection of a traumatic experience. Often the experience recalled is the event that caused the trauma. In other words, the reorganization of the fiber pattern and softening or lengthening of the tissue are sometimes accompanied by the release of associated memory.

Gravity and physical and emotional structure

The ways our lives are influenced by gravity have been thoroughly explored by Rolf in her training and writings (Rolf 1962, 1977). Her work eloquently and scientifically expands upon the concepts of Goldthwait:

◆ Any trauma to the body is recorded as changes in internal structure. With slight damage, structures are nearly able to resume their original positions after healing. But even slight displacements have cumulative and long-term effects, especially if there is a shift in the way weight is carried (a change in the relation to gravity). In fact, it is possible that *all* traumas to the body alter the relation to gravity by causing deviations from the ideal pattern, the form we have inherited to enable us to cope with gravity. Even a small change in alignment and movement will result in compensatory changes throughout the body. Patterns of neural activity, blood and lymph flow, and muscular contraction will be altered. If recovery is prolonged, certain muscles will atrophy from disuse, others will become hypertoned from being overworked. Because muscles act as pumps, moving blood and lymph, the presence of immobilized and flaccid muscles will reduce the nutrition and oxygenation of cells and tissues. When a muscle is chronically shortened, it gradually loses its ability to relax. Tension will always be present. Connective tissue fibrils will be laid down to thicken and strengthen structures that are called upon to provide extra support. Traces of altered structure and function can be retained indefinitely after an injury heals. A widely held misconception in our culture is that these accumulated imbalances, and the discomfort associated with them, are an inevitable effect of ageing, and cannot be reversed. This is not the case.

◆ The way the body responds to physical trauma applies equally to the response to an emotional mishap or to a chronic psychological state. Psychological attitudes are always represented in body structure. Fear, grief, and anger each have a characteristic pose and pattern of movement, sometimes referred to as 'body language' (e.g. Kurtz & Prestera 1976). An emotional response immediately precipitates contraction of flexor muscles and movement away from structural balance. Once this happens, gravity takes over and pulls the structure downward, making the body shorter. Each imbalance must be compensated for by displacements of other parts of the body. Tension and altered function are always present. Recovery from an emotional shock requires flexibility and resiliency of the musculoskeletal system, an ability to return the body toward the ideal pattern of relationship with gravity. If an individual continues to dramatize an emotional situation, the physical body becomes set into a psychological pattern. Once these changes have taken place, the physical attitude becomes invariable, involuntary. Movements, including respiration, reveal the emotional turmoils. In a balanced body, inspiration involves lengthening of the entire spine, from the sacrum all the way up to the cranium. When movements are restricted, individuals can no longer feel an emotion as an emotion. No longer can they have a natural response to an immediate situation and then get on with their life. Instead, they live, move, and have their being in an attitude. No amount of discussion, thought, or mental suggestion can change the pattern. To escape from their chronic fear, grief, or anger, the physical tone of the muscles and the structure in relation to gravity must be changed.

◆ The imbalances resulting from physical or emotional trauma can lead to a whole realm of chronic problems for which conventional medicine has little to offer. The more serious of these, arthritis, high blood pressure, even cancer, are whole-system phenomena that cannot be understood by examining parts rather than relationships. And gravity is a part of the whole that has been given relatively little attention. As an example, consider the relation of the head to gravity. For various reasons, most of us hold our heads tipped forward, with our cervical spine bent. The vertebral artery is curved instead of straight, and its lumen is narrowed, restricting the cervical circulation. Less nourishment reaches the brain and sense organs of the head. The hydrostatic compartments of the brain (ventricles) are affected. The sympathetic–parasympathetic balance can be influenced, leading to digestive complaints. Tensions may lead to headaches and bursitis. The functioning of the spinal cord itself may be impaired at the important region where it descends from the brain. The electric and magnetic fields of the brain and spinal nerves (Ch. 2) may have their patterns distorted by cervical imbalances.

◆ While physical patterns can become solidified from psychological attitudes, the converse is also true. A physical trauma, for example a childhood fall down basement steps, a slip from the bicycle (both a result of gravity), or a devastating motor crash, can influence the emotional state. A relatively simple accident which nevertheless leaves the body malaligned and out of balance can affect the psychological sense of the individual. The kinesthetic body feels inadequate, and the physical structure projects an image of inadequacy.

How can integration within the gravitational field be recognized when it is present? The goal is an organism that is balanced in space around a vertical line (Fig. 11.2E), and that can move with ease and efficiency.

In the next chapter we consider how some therapeutic approaches affect the gravity/movement/energy systems of the body.

References

Bassett C A L 1968 Biologic significance of piezoelectricity. Calcified Tissue Research 1:252–272

Coffey D 1985 See Levine J The man who says YES. Johns Hopkins Magazine (Feb/April): 34–44

Goldthwait J E 1909 The relation of posture to human efficiency and the influence of poise upon the support and function of the viscera. Boston Medical and Surgical Journal 161:839–848

Goldthwait J E 1911 The conservation of human energy: a plea for a broader outlook in the practice of medicine. Rocky Mountain Medical Journal 19(Oct):341–350

Goldthwait J E, Brown L T, Swain L T, Kuhns K G 1934 Body mechanics in the study and treatment of disease. J B Lippincott, Philadelphia

Hellebrandt F A, Franseen E B 1943 Physiological study of the vertical stance of man. Physiological Review 23:220–255

Horwitz A F 1997 Integrins and health: discovered only recently, these adhesive cell surface molecules have quickly revealed themselves to be critical to proper functioning of the body and to life itself. Scientific American 276:68–75

Hyman J M, McLaughlin D W, Scott A C 1981 On Davydov's alpha-helix solution. Physica D 30:23–44

Hynes R O 1992 Integrins: versatility, modulation, and signaling. Cell 69:11–26

Ingber D E 1993a Cellular tensegrity: defining new rules of biological design that govern the cytoskeleton. Journal of Cell Science 104:613–627

Ingber D E 1993b The riddle of morphogenesis: a question of solution chemistry or molecular cell engineering. Cell 75:1249–1252

Ingber D E, Jamieson I 1985 Cells as tensegrity structures. In: Andersson L L, Gahmberg C G, Ekblom P E (eds) Gene expression during normal and malignant differentiation. Academic Press, New York, pp 13–32

Ingber D E, Folkman J 1989 Tension and compression as basic determinants of cell form and function: utilization of a cellular tensegrity mechanism. In: Stein W, Bronner F (eds) Cell shape:

determinants, regulation and regulatory role. Academic Press, San Diego, pp 1–32

Kurtz R, Prestera H 1976 The body reveals. Harper and Row, New York

Lauffenburger D A, Horwitz A F 1996 Cell migration: a physically integrated molecular process. Cell 84:359–396

Myers T W 1997a The 'anatomy trains'. Journal of Bodywork and Movement Therapies 1:91–101

Myers T W 1997b The 'anatomy trains': part 2. Journal of Bodywork and Movement Therapies 1:134–145

Oschman J L 1993 Sensing solitons in soft tissues. Guild News, the news magazine for the Guild for Structural Integration, Boulder, Colorado 3:22–25

Oschman J L, Oschman N H 1994a Somatic recall, part I: soft tissue memory. Massage Therapy Journal, American Massage Therapy Association, Lake Worth, FL, 34:36–45, 111–116

Oschman J L, Oschman N H 1994b Somatic recall, part II: soft tissue holography. Massage Therapy Journal, American Massage Therapy Association, Lake Worth, FL, 34:66–67, 106–110

Pickup A J 1978 Collagen and behaviour: a model for progressive debilitation. International Research Communications System Journal of Medical Science 6:499–502

Pugh A 1976 An introduction to tensegrity. University of California Press, Berkeley

Ratner S 1979 The dynamic state of body proteins. Annals of the New York Academy of Sciences 325:189–209

Robbie D L 1977 Tensional forces in the human body. Orthopaedic Review 6:45–48

Rolf I P 1962 Structural integration. Gravity: an unexplored factor in a more human use of human beings. Journal of the Institute for the Comparative Study of History, Philosophy and the Sciences 1:3–20

Rolf I P 1977 Rolfing: the integration of human structures. Dennis-Landman, Santa Monica, CA

Saleh B E A, Teich N C (eds) 1991 Acousto-optics. In: Fundamentals of Photonics. John Wiley, New York, ch 20, pp 799–831

Schoenheimer R 1942 The dynamic state of

body constituents. Harvard University Press, Cambridge, MA

Strait L A, Inman V T, Ralston H J 1947 Sample illustrations of physical principles selected from physiology and medicine. American Journal of Physiology 15:375–382

Wang J Y, Butler J P, Ingber D E 1993 Mechanotransduction across the cell surface and through the cytoskeleton. Science 260:1124–1127

Warwick R, Williams P L 1973 Gray's anatomy, 35th [British] edn. Churchill Livingstone, Edinburgh

Weiss P 1961 The biological foundation of wound repair. Harvey Lectures 55:13–42

Wolff J 1892 Das Gesetz der Transformation der Knochen. A Hirschwald, Berlin

Young J Z 1957 The life of mammals. Oxford University Press, New York

12 Structural integration (Rolfing®), osteopathic, chiropractic, Feldenkrais, Alexander, myofascial release, and related methods

Introduction

Awareness of the biology of gravity has always been implicit in approaches ranging from physical therapy, kinesiology, yoga, chiropractic, osteopathy, Alexander, Feldenkrais, as well as gait analysis, furniture design and construction of prosthetic limbs, to name a few.

The basic principle of gravitational biology is known to any child who plays with blocks. The centre of gravity of each block must be vertically above the centre of gravity of the one below, to have a stable, balanced arrangement. If the centre of gravity of one block lies outside of the gravity line, stability is compromised.

Likewise, there is only one stable, strain-free arrangement of the parts of the human body. Any variation from this orientation will require corresponding compensations in other parts of the support system. Goldthwait, Rolf, and others have written eloquently about this perspective.

Rolf was aware of Goldthwait's research (Asher, personal communication, 1990), and concurred that misalignment of any part will affect the whole system, and that restoration of verticality is a way to address a wide variety of clinical problems.

Many therapists know intuitively, or from their training, that physical and personality structure are intimately related. Rolf and her colleagues have documented the relationship between structural, kinetic and emotional stability.

The 'stack of blocks' analogy is limited, because the body is broader at the top than at the base, and because the body can move about. Balance is not static but dynamic. Moreover, blocks are designed only to resist compression. Buckminster Fuller's contribution was to explain how nature uses tension as well as compression to create stable yet movable structures.

Rolf took the next step by discerning within the body a fundamental pattern or inherited form that is specifically designed to enable us to function in the gravity field. It is a form in which each anatomical part and each function is supported by the parts and functions below it. It is a dynamic form. Hence, for any movement, there is a pattern of tensions and compressions that is economical, efficient, graceful and precise. Optimal performance occurs only at the narrow peak of balance. This is the pattern that seems most aesthetically satisfying. The slightest deviation alerts us. Balanced motion is beautiful and effective. The grace and ease of integrated activity motivates us to attend the athletic event, ballet or any other artistic performance.

Perfect movement is rare in a world in which our physical and emotional bodies are subject to many kinds of interference. Even at the Olympic Games, perfection is rare, and it stands out, and thrills us when we see it. Experience shows that even the most intense training does not liberate the performer from all of the restrictions to movement. Hands-on bodywork and movement therapies can extend range and efficiency of motion, flexibility, resiliency, balance, timing, precision. To this mix, Rolf added another essential ingredient: emotional integration. And there is still more to the story.

While effortless coordination and aesthetic appeal are valued, and dynamic emotional stability is essential to achieving and sustaining them, there is a broader significance to the balancing and integration of human structures. Muscular balance is the outward and visible sign that vital communications and energy flows are functioning freely. By communications, we are referring to the flow of body fluids, the flow of neural impulses and the flow of vibrations through the semiconducting tensegrous living matrix. These are the vibrations that convey the information needed for the support system to adapt itself to the way it is being used, and to repair injuries. In a balanced and communicating body, various kinds of vibratory information percolate throughout the body and into every cell and nucleus.

One way of defining energy is from physics: the ability to do work. When muscular efficiency is optimal, the expenditure of energy by the body in any activity – working, walking, running, or whatever – is minimal. Hence there is more energy available for other vital functions such as thought, digestion, circulation, tissue maintenance, repair, defense against disease, etc. Along with this greater efficiency comes a greater psychological ease and emotional security. The integrated body not only accomplishes a multitude of tasks, but it carries them out simultaneously, effortlessly, joyously.

Joint alignment

Manipulative therapies, such as osteopathy and chiropractic, recognize the importance of joint alignment in the health of the nervous system. Some schools employ the concept of 'vital force' flowing through the healthy joint, while others do not refer to life energy in order to avoid the historical biases and controversies documented in Chapter 1. The vital force is usually associated with the flow of nerve impulses, and a misaligned joint interferes with this flow. The fundamental unit of disturbance is called the subluxation (Fig. 12.1A). Much research has been done on the effects of subluxations on physiological processes (e.g. Aguayo et al 1971). The subluxation concept can be expanded to include other energetic aspects of joint alignment. We have described the fibrous systems in the connective tissue as a semiconductor communication network, and this applies to the collagenous fibers running through the vertebrae and the intervertebral discs (Fig. 12.1B). Hence alignment influences two kinds of communication: nerve impulses and semiconduction through the tensegrous network. These considerations apply to the fibers spanning any joint in the body (e.g. Fig. 12.1C).

Alignment of the collagenous networks has consequences for the overall energy field of the body (Fig. 12.2A). As discussed in Chapter 4, the overall shape of this field corresponds to that of a coil or solenoid with electricity flowing through it (Fig. 12.2B). The main source of the electricity in the body is the electric field of the heart. The primary set of vertical conductors giving rise to the overall biomagnetic field consists of the muscles and connective tissues associated with the spine and the large blood vessels.

The collagenous fibers of connective tissue are actually triple helices (Fig. 12.2C). From the perspective of electronic circuitry, there are three different ways of connecting coils together: in series (Fig. 12.2D), in parallel (Fig. 12.2E) and in series-parallel (Fig. 12.2F). The series parallel arrangement best describes the arrangement in the connective tissue system of the body.

In terms of the magnetic fluxes through the vertebral column and surrounding tissues which give rise to the overall field of the body, the best arrangement is one in which the axes of the fibers are parallel and in alignment (Fig. 12.2G). Departures from the parallel arrangement (Fig. 12.2H) will tend to reduce the total magnetic flux through the system and thereby reduce the strength of the overall field.

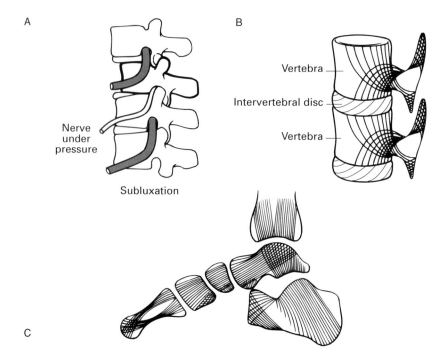

Fig. 12.1 **A** The fundamental unit of disorder in chiropractic and osteopathic approaches is the subluxation, in which nerve function is compromised by pressure exerted by misaligned bones. **B** Connective tissue fibers extend from vertebrae through the intervertebral disc. It is proposed here that an additional aspect of the subluxation is the disturbance in alignment of connective tissue fibers through the joint. **C** A good example of the importance of alignment of fibers in joints is provided by the anatomy of the foot. (From Thompson 1992, Fig. 464, p. 980 and used with the publisher's permission.)

Plasticity and energy flows

A consequence of this point of view is that every joint in the body participates in the energy flows essential to life, and that alignment depends on both the position of the hard tissues (bone) and the arrangement of the surrounding soft tissues (ligaments and tendons). While manipulative therapies focus on bony alignment and elimination of subluxations, deep tissue methods such as structural integration or Rolfing® emphasize the properties of the soft tissues, and the opening of 'myofascial constrictions'. There are several techniques and mechanisms by which deep tissue work affects soft tissues. One was suggested by Rolf (1977):

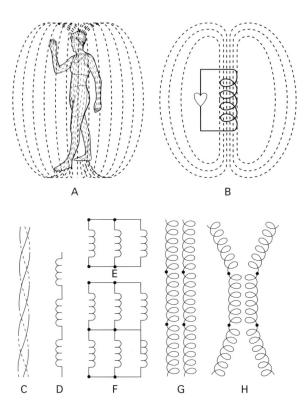

Fig. 12.2 **A** The overall field of the body. **B** The field shown in **A** is generated primarily by the flow of electricity generated by the heart. The currents flow mainly through the muscles and connective tissue fibers associated with the spine. **C** The connective tissue fibers (collagen) are triple helices. From the perspective of electronic circuitry, the arrangement of connective tissue fibers can be described as in series **D**, in parallel **E**, or, most appropriately, series-parallel **F**. In view of this arrangement of collagen and other helical molecules, it is logical that the field will be enhanced when the helices are parallel **G** rather than out of alignment **H**.

While fascia is characteristically a tissue of collagen fibers, these must be visualized as embedded in ground substance. For the most part, the latter is an amorphous semifluid gel. The collagen fibers are demonstrably slow to change and are a definite chemical entity. Therefore, the speed so clearly apparent in fascial change (plasticity) must be a property of its complex ground substance. The universal distribution of connective tissue calls attention to the likelihood that this colloidal gel is the universal internal environment. Every living cell seems to be in contact with it, and its modification under changes of pressure would account for the wide spectrum

of effects seen in Structural Integration (Rolfing®). The observable speed of
the changes that are induced supports this hypothesis in the light of what we
know about the action of colloids and the physical laws governing them.
The application of pressure is, in fact, the addition of energy to the tissue
colloid. (It is well-known in physics that the addition of energy can turn
colloid gel into sol.) It is probably this more energized colloid that accounts
for the different physical properties of the body undergoing Structural
Integration. (Rolf 1977)

That such changes can take place has been known for a long time. Figure 12.3
shows how pressure changes the viscosity of an organic gel (Brown 1934a,b;
Brown & Marsland 1936; Marsland & Brown 1942). The cytoplasmic matrix is
a labile gel, as it is held together with weak bonds. It can dissolve rapidly upon
application of a shearing force, such as would result from pressure. The striking feature is the great speed with which solation can occur when pressure is
applied, and the speed with which the matrix re-gels after the pressure is released.
Indeed, the cytoplasmic matrix falls apart normally during mitosis, and re-
forms after the chromosomes have segregated into the two daughter cells.

Research on gels has confirmed that they are highly labile, and has shown that
other forces, such as electrical fields and heat, can bring about the gel-to-sol
transition (Tanaka 1981). Other work (Reddy & Cochran 1979) has shown that
application of pressure results in a flow of interstitial fluids and ground
substance away from a region under pressure. If stress, disuse and lack of

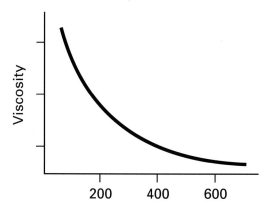

Fig. 12.3 The effect of pressure on the viscosity of an organic gel (the
cytoplasmic ground substance of amoeba and sea urchin). (After Brown
and Marsland 1936, Fig. 3, p. 142, with permission of the Journal of
Cellular and Comparative Physiology.)

movement cause the gel to dehydrate, contract and harden (an idea that is supported both by scientific evidence and by the experiences of many somato-therapists) the application of pressure seems to bring about a rapid solation and rehydration. Removal of the pressure allows the system to rapidly re-gel, but in the process the tissue is transformed, both in its water content and in its ability to conduct energy and movement. The ground substance becomes more porous, a better medium for the diffusion of nutrients, oxygen, waste products of metabolism, and the enzymes and building-blocks involved in the 'metabolic regeneration' process elucidated by Schoenheimer (Fig. 12.4).

Release of toxins

Another effect of the gel-to-sol and return-to-gel transitions is the release of toxins that have been trapped in the sponge-like interstices of the ground substance. It is likely that toxins and metabolic waste products can accumulate in connective tissues, particularly in areas that have become densified as a response to trauma or structural imbalance. The process is called 'storage excretion'. The connective tissue gel can trap materials both mechanically (because of the small channels between its fibers) and electrically (because of its abundant negative charges). Pressure releases these trapped materials, some of which may have been stored for many years. They are released into the interstitial fluid and carried away by the lymphatic and venous drainage, and are excreted.

At the same time, the application of pressure to the myofascial system produces piezoelectric fields and streaming potentials that stimulate the surrounding cells. The strength of these fields in a particular tissue depends upon the angle with which the pressure is applied.

Mechanisms

A mechanism to explain how the gel-to-sol-to-gel transformation can quickly bring the body back into anatomical balance is shown in Figure 12.5. As a response to a chronic structural or emotional imbalance, connective tissue fibers bunch-up, forming dense regions at the ends of tendons and ligaments where they attach to bones (Fig. 12.5A). This 'kinking' of the collagen bundles shortens the tendon or ligament, tenses the muscles and strains joints. Lack of motion and poor circulation to these dense regions leads to dehydration and shrinking of the ground substance. Cells become energetically isolated from the living matrix system. Photomicrographs of crimped or kinked patterns in collagen fibers in ligaments have been published (Frank and Shrive 1995).

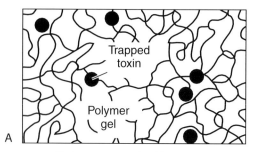

Polymer network with trapped
toxins

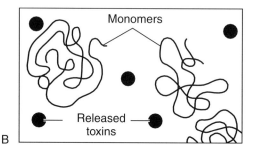

Depolymerized network
releases toxins

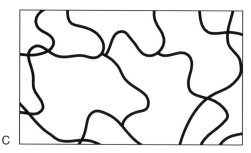

Repolymerized network

Fig. 12.4 Proposed scheme for the effect of pressure on the gel phase (ground substance) of connective tissue. **A** A dehydrated gel with trapped particles (dots) such as toxic substances. **B** The application of pressure converts the gel to a sol, releasing trapped particles which are carried away by the lymphatic and venous drainage, to be processed by the excretory system. **C** When pressure is removed the ground substance re-gels, but it is now more porous, open, hydrated, and free of toxic materials which have been processed by the excretory system.

The immediate effect of pressure is to soften these dense kinked regions, allowing the tendon or ligament to lengthen, and enabling chronically tightened muscles to relax, as shown in Figure 12.5B. While this idea has not been tested directly, it does provide a possible explanation for one of the immediate effects of deep tissue work. When all of the tendons and ligaments in the body have been treated appropriately, the individual can become taller, more relaxed and more balanced. Physical and emotional insecurities resolve.

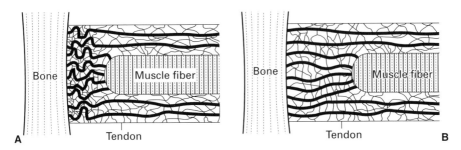

Fig. 12.5 A Kinking of collagen fibers at the ends of tendons could be caused by dehydration of ground substance. **B** Application of pressure (as in Structural Integration or Rolfing®) may cause temporary solation of the ground substance, permitting kinked collagen fibrils to lengthen, allowing chronically shortened muscles to relax, and reducing strain on joints.

Another mechanism that accounts for rapid changes in body structure produced during Rolfing®, Feldenkrais, Alexander, osteopathic, craniosacral therapy, yoga stretching, movement therapies and other methods, involves effects on the neural feedback systems that regulate muscle tone. The receptors in this system include the Golgi tendon organs, which are located in the muscle insertions. Methods that actively stretch these areas can change muscle tone throughout the body and increase the overall integration of neuromuscular balance (e.g. Cottingham 1985).

Some conclusions

From the information summarized here, it can be seen why the way individuals stand and move gives a detailed history of their physical and emotional life. Body shape and patterns of movement simultaneously tell three stories, each relating to the way we experience gravity:

◆ An evolutionary history, representing the millions of years that our ancestors adapted to life in the gravity field of our planet

◆ A shorter history of personal traumas and adaptations during our lifetime

◆ The story of our present emotional state, including the effects of our most recent experiences.

Previous chapters have focused on the wealth of energy and information flows that allow the various parts of the body to work together at all levels: systems, organs, tissues, cells and nuclei. Theory and practice indicate that any therapy that brings the visible parts of the body into alignment, or that restores flexibility and mobility, will, at the same time, facilitate vital communications and thereby have beneficial effects upon the health of the fascial supporting systems. Once the body has been organized around the vertical, and dynamic movements have become optimized, 'gravity becomes the therapist' (Rolf 1977).

References

Aguayo A, Nair CPV, Midgley R 1971 Experimental progressive compression neuropathy in the rabbit. Archives of Neurology 24: 359–364

Brown DES 1934a The pressure coefficient of 'viscosity' in the eggs of *Arbacia punctulata*. Journal of Cellular and Comparative Physiology 5:335–346

Brown DES 1934b The effect of rapid changes in hydrostatic pressure upon the contraction of skeletal muscle. Journal of Cellular and Comparative Physiology 4: 257– 281

Brown DES, Marsland DA 1936 The viscosity of amoeba at high hydrostatic pressure. Journal of Cellular and Comparative Physiology 8:159–165

Cottingham JT 1985 Healing through touch. Rolf Institute, Boulder, Colorado. Ch. 16

Frank CB, Shrive NG 1995 Ligament. In: Nigg BM, Herzog W (eds)

Biomechanics of the Musculo-Skeletal System. John Wiley, Chicester, ch 2.3, Fig 2.3.2, p 110

Marsland DA, Brown DES 1942 The effects of pressure on sol-gel equilibria, with special reference to myosin and other protoplasmic gels. Journal of Cellular and Comparative Physiology 20: 295–305

Reddy NP, Cochran G Van B 1979 Phenomenological theory underlying pressure-time relationship in decubitus ulcer formation. Federation Proceedings 38: 1153 (abstract no. 4885)

Rolf IP 1977 Rolfing: The Integration of Human Structures. Dennis-Landman, Santa Monica, CA

Tanaka T 1981 Gels. Scientific American 244: 124–138

Thompson D'W 1992 On growth and form. Dover Publications, New York (first published 1942)

13 The electromagnetic environment

Introduction

To complete our presentation, it is important to consider both the beneficial and the potentially harmful effects of electromagnetic radiation present in our environment. Some of these forms of energy are produced by technology, and others are related to geophysical and meteorological phenomena that are not widely known to the public. To what extent do these energies complement or interfere with the delicate and intricate electrical and electronic signaling systems that regulate vital biological processes? Can these energies enhance or compromise the nurturing environment of the therapeutic setting? What do patients need to know about this subject to get the most benefit from their therapies?

This chapter examines the sources of energy fields in the environment and the responsiveness of living systems to them. Historical detail is included to help the reader understand that there is an extensive literature on these subjects. Some of this literature is very reliable, some is completely outdated. Chapter 14 focuses on the potential harmful effects of environmental fields, and what can be done about them.

Biology and physics at odds

Biologists have repeatedly documented the great sensitivity organisms have to exceedingly tiny signals in their environment. A host of sensory systems are employed for a variety of survival purposes. Organisms use energetic cues to locate and orient themselves geographically, to set their biological rhythms, to detect prey, predators, and mates, and to anticipate meteorological and earth changes, including seasonal variations, weather fronts, hurricanes, tornadoes, and earthquakes (Presman 1970, Dubrov 1978, Ho et al 1994).

Extreme examples of energy sensitivity have been discovered for virtually all living systems at all levels of organization: bacteria, algae, higher plants, protozoa, flatworms, insects such as honeybees, snails, fish, birds such as carrier pigeons, green turtles, sharks, whales, and humans (summarized by Kalmijn 1971, Adey & Bawin 1977, Warnke 1994).

For several decades, physics seemed to be at odds with these discoveries. Physicists treat living systems like other forms of matter. Known or measurable properties of cells and tissues and the established laws of electricity and magnetism are employed to calculate the currents induced in tissues by environmental fields of various sorts. The calculations are based on the degree that fields of different frequencies penetrate into the body, tissue conductivity, viscosity and dielectric properties, interactions of induced currents with larger currents from other sources, the 'noise' from random thermal agitation at body temperature, and so on. A consistent conclusion is that environmental fields can have no biological effects on living matter unless the energy intensity is sufficient to ionize or heat tissues (e.g. Foster & Guy 1986, Foster & Pickard 1987, Wachtel 1995). Weaker fields may induce microcurrents in living tissues, but these are millions of times smaller than the noise from thermal agitation and normal physiological signaling processes, and should therefore have no biological effects. The biology must be wrong.

The dilemma resolved

This physics/biology dilemma was resolved when careful research revealed that biological systems completely defy a simple and obvious logic: larger stimuli should produce larger responses. In living systems extremely weak fields may have potent effects, while there may be little or no response to strong fields. A turning point in the controversy came about when scientists from the prestigious Neurosciences Research Program examined the evidence, and concluded that:

> a striking range of biological interactions has been described in experiments where control procedures appear to have been adequately considered . . .
> The existence of biological effects of very weak electromagnetic fields suggests an extraordinarily efficient mechanism for detecting these fields and discriminating them from much higher levels of noise. The underlying mechanisms must necessarily involve ever increasing numbers of elements in the sensing system, ordered in particular ways to form a cooperative organization and manifesting similar forms and levels of energy over long distances. (Adey & Bawin 1977)

This statement signaled the emergence of a new paradigm in biology that has led to extensive research and clinical investigation into the beneficial and harmful effects of electromagnetic fields. We now know that cells and tissues are highly non-linear, non-equilibrium, cooperative, and coherent systems, capable of responding to very specific 'windows' (Fig.13.1) in terms of frequency and intensity (Adey 1990).

Clinical applications

Biomedical researchers have been testing the use of pulsing magnetic fields originating outside the organism to induce microcurrents within tissues to stimulate healing (see Ch. 6). A consistent observation is that triggering a cellular response requires the application of energy in a very narrow range of frequencies and intensities (Bassett 1978, 1995). Extensive research on fracture non-unions led to the statement that, 'jump starting a car with a dead battery creates an operational machine; exposure of a nonunion to PEMFs can convert

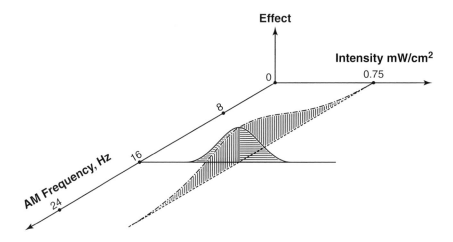

Fig. 13.1 A frequency-power window. The frequency-power-density 'window' or 'response surface' for the brain. The measured response was calcium ion efflux from chick forebrain tissue. The fundamental signal frequency was 147 MHz (million cycles per second). This signal was amplitude modulated sinusoidally at selected frequencies and power densities. This study, published by Blackman and colleagues (1979) confirmed earlier work by Bawin et al (1975) who reported that brain tissue has a maximum frequency sensitivity in the ELF range, between 6 and 20 Hz and intensity of 10^{-7} V/cm. This is the level associated with navigation and prey detection in marine vertebrates and with control of human biological rhythms. The amplitude modulated microwave signal has an intensity window around 10^{-1} V/cm. This is at the level of the electroencephalogram (EEG) in brain tissue (see also Adey 1980). (After Blackman et al 1979, Fig. 4, p. 97, with permission from Modern Radio Science, the International Union of Radio Science and the American Geophysical Union.)

a stalled healing process to active repair, even in patients unhealed for as long as 40 years!' (Bassett 1995).

Microampere currents induced from outside the body restart the healing process by recruiting bone-forming cells in a manner similar to a natural repair response. Field effects are highly specific and confined to a narrow power frequency window. Too high an induced current stimulates tissue necrosis rather than repair. And the characteristics of a 'bone healing pulse' are different from those of an 'osteonecrosis pulse'.

Oschman (1997a) noted the similarity between the frequencies and intensities of low energy emissions from the hands of therapists and the signals from pulsed electromagnetic field (PEMF) devices used in clinical medicine. Medical researchers have documented a cascade of signal transduction processes from the cell membrane to the nucleus and on to the genetic material that are facilitated by PEMF therapies (Bassett 1995). Polarity, Reiki, therapeutic touch, acupuncture, and many hands-on therapies probably affect the same signal pathways. Evidence presented in the next chapter will describe how electromagnetic pollution at somewhat higher frequencies (50 or 60 Hz) appears to have negative effects on the same pathways (see Ch. 14).

Mechanisms

Much is being learned about the biophysical mechanisms involved in the amplification of tiny signals to produce significant physiological and behavioral effects (e.g. Ho et al 1994, Oschman 2000). All of this information has relevance to energy therapists who wish to validate and explain their experiences.

Biologists accept that living molecules exist in the context of a myriad of violent and random thermal fluctuations. Yet cells and tissues and organs must maintain their precise and intricate actions and reactions, responses and adjustments, unperturbed by the thermal noise. In order to survive, living systems have developed a variety of tricks to get around the more obvious physical limits to sensitivity.

Of particular importance in understanding the physical mechanisms involved was the realization that molecular 'sensors' in living systems are actually highly ordered arrays of molecules. These are the 'ever increasing numbers of elements in the sensing system, ordered in particular ways to form a cooperative organization and manifesting similar forms and levels of energy over long distances' mentioned in the Adey & Bawin (1977) quotation above.

Fröhlich and others have described the physics and sensitivity of molecular arrays in great detail (Fröhlich 1968a, 1968b, 1970, 1974, 1975, 1988; Ho 1998). Fröhlich focused on the arrays of phospholipid molecules in cell membranes, but there are many other arrays in living tissues (Fig. 13.3). All of these are electrically polarized and are probable components of the sensing apparatus:

◆ Arrays of phospholipid molecules in cell membranes

◆ Collagen arrays in connective tissues

◆ Arrays of chlorophyll molecules in the leaf

◆ Myelin sheaths of nerves

◆ Contractile arrays in muscles

◆ Arrays of sensory endings in the retina

◆ Arrays of microtubules, microfilaments, and other fibrous components of the cytoskeleton in nerves and other kinds of cells, including the cilia of sensory organs such as those responsible for detecting odors, sounds, and gravity (the vestibular apparatus).

In general, organisms are poised to respond to minute 'whispers' in the electromagnetic environment. Bassett (1995) suggested a fascinating analogy between the *arrays* of bone cells in the osteon and the *phased arrays* of radio telescope antennas, such as those at Jodrell Bank in Cheshire, England (Fig. 13.2). Radio telescope arrays enable astrophysicists to detect extremely weak electromagnetic signals from nebulae thousands of millions of light years away. Bassett suggested that tissues extract information from fields originating outside the body by a physical process akin to that involved in radio astronomy (Fig. 13.2). It seems to this author (Oschman 2000) that the collagen and mineral arrays of the bone probably serve as the antenna array, while the cellular osteon contains the electronic solid state circuitry that detects and interprets the information contained in electromagnetic fields. This hypothetical concept could apply to all of the cellular and tissue arrays listed above and shown in Figure 13.3. Note that these arrays make up much of the structural features of the living organism.

The physical mechanisms suggested by Fröhlich and by Bassett are not the only models that have been proposed. Other concepts are described by Bridges & Preache (1981), by Lednev (1991), and by Liboff (1985).

Biosensors

We now examine some of the specific sensory systems found in nature:

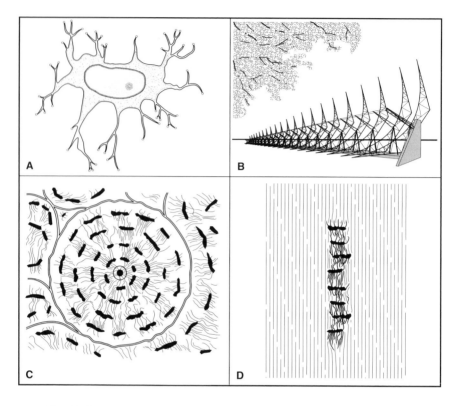

Fig. 13.2 Bone compared to a radio-telescope array. Bassett (1995) made the analogy between the array of osteocytes in the osteon and the phased radio telescope array. **A** Shows a single osteocyte. There is a central nucleus and a large number of slender processes or extensions of the cell surface. **B** A phased array of radio-telescope antennas such as those at Jodrell Bank in England. (Redrawn from Hoyle 1962, p. 202, and used with kind permission from Sir Fred Hoyle.) **C** An osteon, the cylindrical unit of compact bone. Each osteon has a blood vessel running through its center, and this is surrounded by an array of electrically interconnected osteocytes. (Adapted with permission from Bassett 1995, copyright © 1995, American Chemical Society.) **D** The osteon is embedded in another array composed of collagen molecules. These are precisely offset, like the elements of a radio telescope array.

The retina

The most remarkable and thoroughly studied sensor in the human body is the eye. The retina contains a protein, rhodopsin, which absorbs light. Careful research, which is still in progress, is showing how the rhodopsin molecule is designed for its task. Energy is stored within its structure in such a way that a single photon can activate a large shift in molecular structure. This shift triggers

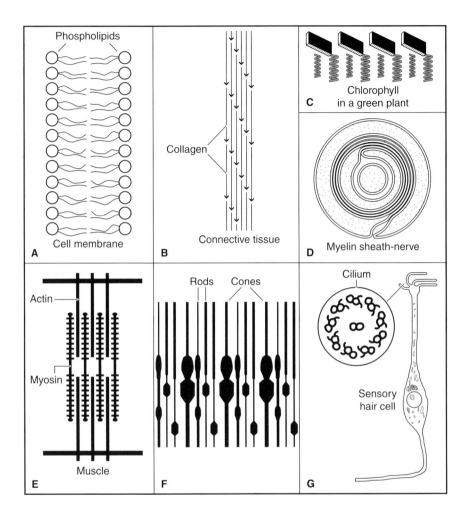

Fig. 13.3 Crystalline arrays in living systems. Crystalline arrangements are the rule and not the exception in living systems. **A** Arrays of phospholipid molecules form cell membranes. **B** Collagen arrays form connective tissue. **C** Arrays of chlorophyll molecules in the leaf. **D** The myelin sheath of nerves. **E** The contractile array in muscle is composed of actin and myosin molecules organized around each other. **F** The array of sensory endings in the retina. **G** Arrays of microtubules, microfilaments, and other fibrous components of the cytoskeleton occur in nerves and other kinds of cells. The example shown here is the cilia of sensory organs such as those responsible for detecting odors and sound. (Illustration **D** is reproduced with permission of Arnold.)

a cascade of chemical reactions, the flow of millions of sodium ions across the rod cell membrane, and an electrical signal that is transmitted by the optic nerves to the brain. In essence, the absorption of each photon is amplified many times to produce a nerve impulse (Stryer 1985, 1987, 1988).

Other senses

The retina is just one of the sensory systems that enable the organism to build up an accurate image and awareness of itself in relation to its surroundings. The traditional five senses are sight, hearing, smell, taste, and touch. However, it is obvious that there are other senses besides the traditional five. Murchie (1978) lists 32. As an example, some people can 'hear' radar, an electromagnetic signal in the microwave region of the electromagnetic spectrum (Guy et al 1975). An ability to detect cosmic rays with the eye has been documented (D'Arcy & Porter 1962, Wick 1972). There is discussion of whether or not these sensory systems are also able to respond to a single quantum of energy, as the retina appears to be able to do (Bialek 1987).

The natural electromagnetic energy spectrum

Geomagnetism

Geomagnetism is far more widely researched than most people realize. In 1940, Chapman & Bartels wrote a 1000 page book that collected and reviewed some 100 000 pages of printed matter on the subject. In 1967, 27 years later, Matsushita & Campbell (1967) edited a two-volume work that attempted to cover the enormous amount of new literature that followed the earlier review. By 1987, four volumes, written by more than 25 authors, were required to treat the phenomenally growing area of research (Jacobs 1987). A bimonthly journal, *Geomagnetism and Aeronomy*, was begun in 1961, and continues to publish research articles on the ionosphere, geomagnetism, and atmospheric radio noise.

Geomagnetic variations

The magnetic field of the earth, called the geomagnetic field, causes the compass needle to point toward the North Pole. However, if you look carefully at a compass needle with a microscope, you will see that the needle is rarely still – it dances back and forth in a variety of rhythms.

◆ Oscillations of the compass needle were first observed by the great London clockmaker George Graham. In 1722 and 1723, Graham made over 1000 observations of the compass declination at his house on Fleet Street (Graham 1724). He observed the declination at different times during the day, using three 12-in compasses that had delicate pivots and fine graduations so that the slightest movements could be detected. He noted that 'all of the needles . . . would not only vary in their direction on different days but at different times on the same day, and this difference would sometimes amount to upwards of 30' in one day, sometimes in a few hours'.

◆ These results were confirmed by Celsius and Hiorter in Uppsala, Sweden, during the period 1740–47. On the clear night of March 1, 1741, Hiorter noticed a large oscillation of the needle, through several degrees, in sympathy with the northern lights or aurora borealis (quoted by Hansteen 1819). In the same year (1741) Celsius and Graham collaborated to determine if the compass variations occurred simultaneously in different places. On April 5, 1741, the magnetic needle at London had an unusual motion at the same time that a disturbance of nearly 2° was recorded in Uppsala. Alexander von Humboldt termed these disturbances 'magnetic storms' (see Malin 1987).

◆ On quiet, undisturbed days there are still variations in the direction of north. Geomagnetic rhythms range in frequency from moment-to-moment to millions of years. The rhythmic variations over the past 4 million years have been documented by studying magnetic minerals in deep-sea sediments collected by drilling core samples (Valet & Meynadier 1993).

◆ In the late 1830s, von Humboldt, in collaboration with Gauss, formed the Göttingen Magnetic Union to organize the data from observatories that maintained records of the magnetic variations. Intensive observations were made on certain days each year. The results were published in six *Annual Reports of the Magnetic Union* (1836–41).

◆ By 1987, there were some 150 magnetic observatories around the world. Here the direction of the magnetic field is monitored continuously using a variometer, and recorded on a magnetogram. A light beam is reflected from a mirror attached to the compass, and focused onto a sheet of photographic paper on a drum rotating once per day. The recorded data are tabulated, sent to World Data centers, and published in yearbooks that are distributed to libraries around the world (see Wienert [1970]).

Some of the geomagnetic rhythms are diurnal (24 hour), some are much slower, and others are quite fast, in the extremely low frequency (ELF) range in the electromagnetic spectrum. The last are now called geomagnetic micropulsations. They are caused by a unique geophysical mechanism known as the Schumann resonance.

Schumann resonance

As mentioned above, the biological effects of natural energy fields are being carefully researched. An important geophysical phenomenon, the Schumann resonance, provides a physical link between solar, lunar, planetary, and other celestial rhythms and human physiology (see also Ch. 7).

In the 1950s, a German atmospheric physicist, W. O. Schumann, suggested that the space between the surface of the earth and the ionosphere should act as a resonant cavity, somewhat like the chamber in a musical instrument.

What do we mean by a resonant cavity? Pressing the keys on a wind instrument changes the size of the air space or cavity, and therefore changes the frequency of the standing waves within that cavity. Standing waves are produced when waves traveling in the cavity are reflected from its boundaries. Each reflection gives rise to a wave traveling in the opposite direction. The reflected waves are superimposed on the original waves to produce what are called *standing waves*. Figure 13.4 shows what is meant by standing waves and resonant cavities in musical instruments and in the atmosphere. Organs use pipes of different sizes to produce standing waves of different frequencies. Pressing a guitar or violin string against the fret or fingerboard changes the effective length of the string and therefore the resonant frequency of the standing waves that can be produced.

Resonant tones are generated when the musician blows over an orifice or past a vibrating reed, or plucks or bows a string. Energy for the Schumann resonance is provided by cloud-to-ground lightning (Fig. 13.4). While you may be experiencing calm weather where you are now, there are, on average, hundreds of lightning strikes taking place each second, some 40 million per day, scattered about the planet. To use the physics terminology, lightning *pumps* energy into the earth–ionosphere cavity, and causes it to vibrate or resonate at frequencies in the ELF range.

In a series of papers published between 1952 and 1957, Schumann gradually refined his resonance theory (see Sentman 1995 for references). In 1954, Schumann and König detected the resonances (Schumann & König 1954). After the initial reports, there followed a period of intense research (1965–82), stimulated in part by the US Navy, which was interested in studying the extremely low frequency band for use in communicating with submerged submarines.

Lightning creates electromagnetic standing waves that travel around the globe at the speed of light. These waves circumnavigate the entire planet on average 7.86 times per second. Hence an observer at any point on the earth's surface will experience both the high frequency electromagnetic signals from the lightning and the extremely low frequency pulsations generated by the atmospheric standing waves. The high frequency waves are reflected from the

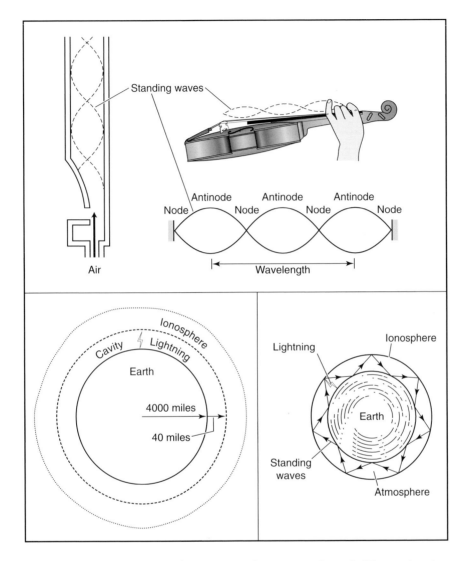

Fig. 13.4 Standing waves and resonances. Organs use pipes of different sizes to produce different notes. Pressing a guitar or violin string against the fret or fingerboard changes the effective length of the string and therefore the resonant frequency of the standing waves that can be produced. Energy for the Schumann resonance is provided by cloud-to-ground lightning. To use the physics terminology, lightning *pumps* energy into the earth–ionosphere cavity, and causes it to vibrate or resonate at frequencies in the ELF range. Lightning creates electromagnetic standing waves that travel around the globe at the speed of light. These waves circumnavigate the entire planet on average 7.86 times per second. The high frequency waves are reflected from the ionosphere, back to the earth, back to the ionosphere, etc. This 'skip' phenomenon has been widely studied, because it is the basis for long distance radio communication. (The diagram at lower right is modified from Bentar 1976, Fig. 15, p. 90, with kind permission of Integral Publishing.)

ionosphere, back to the earth, back to the ionosphere, etc. (Fig. 13.4). This 'skip' phenomenon has been widely studied, because it is the basis for long distance radio communication.

As electromagnetic waves, the low frequency Schumann micropulsations can be detected either as electric or as magnetic fields. The average frequency is about 7–10 Hz, and this corresponds to the average frequency of brain waves in humans. This correlation is thought to have evolutionary and physiological significance (e.g. Direnfeld 1983, Becker 1990). When the ionosphere gets higher – on the night side of the planet, for example – the cavity gets larger, and the resonant frequency drops. Rhythms of terrestrial and extraterrestrial origin alter the height and other properties of the ionosphere, and thereby alter the Schumann frequency in the range of 1–40 Hz. There are also variations in the global lightning frequency. There are times when solar activity leads to magnetic storms that disrupt the ionosphere, and Schumann resonances cease completely.

To summarize, the Schumann resonance is created by terrestrial phenomena, and is modified or modulated by extraterrestrial activities. A thorough and technical review of the literature on the Schumann resonance has been published by Sentman (1995).

VLF-sferics

In addition to its role in 'pumping' energy into the atmosphere, to maintain the Schumann resonance, lightning directly produces a variety of signals in the very low frequency (VLF) range (1–100 kHz). These are called VLF-atmospherics or VLF-sferics. Sferics are impulses that propagate at about the speed of light through the atmosphere. The signals gradually become dispersed and damped with distance, and higher and lower frequency components are lost, leaving a signal of about 10 kHz. At distances beyond 1000 km, the 10 kHz signal predominates (Schienle et al 1998).

Other extraterrestrial sources

In addition to the Schumann resonance and the sferics, the surface of the earth is exposed to a variety of other extraterrestrial electromagnetic signals, including X-rays and cosmic rays. Volland (1984) is a good source of information on this subject.

We have described the Schumann resonance and VLF-sferics because they are the phenomena most widely studied for their possible biological effects.

Geopathic stress

Finally, it is important to mention the important concept of geopathic stress. A number of investigators have identified 'earth radiations' that occur at particular 'pathogenic sites' that can be detected by dowsing. While some scientists regard both geopathic stress and dowsing as lunatic fringe, others have seriously explored the phenomena involved.

It appears that underground fluid flows, as in springs or pipes, can create a kind of field. Where water and/or electric currents flow at different depths, and cross each other, interference patterns are set up. Some of these can be beneficial, others appear to be harmful.

Research on this subject was begun in 1922 in Central Europe following a study of unusually high cancer death rates in the German town of Vilsbiburg. Physicians compared the medical records with maps created by dowsers. There was a correlation between geopathic stress zones and serious illness (von Pohl 1985). A 1989 study in Austria yielded similar results. The importance of this phenomenon is widely recognized in Germany, where efforts are made to keep health records on individual homes (Best 1988). This literature is summarized by Smith & Best (1989) and by Miller (1998).

Some clinicians can identify signs of geopathic stress in their cancer patients, and regard the information as essential to their treatments. 'Pathogenic sites' can be identified both by dowsing and with sensitive magnetometers. It is particularly important that one's bed not be located above a geopathic zone (Fig. 13.5). Spending many hours a day in such a region can affect the body's energetic communication systems, compromise the immune system, and lead to serious disease (Aschoff 1986). In Britain, the Dulwich Health Society has documented case histories and published methods of assessing and preventing geopathic stress (Gordon 1988).

The energy spectrum of technology

It is only within the last 100 years that electricity has become abundantly available throughout much of the world. This has led to the evolution of the enormous range of devices, appliances, and technologies that we take for granted, seldom appreciating that none of this existed but a short time ago. The 'filling in' of the electromagnetic spectrum over the last century is dramatically illustrated by Figure 13.6. In a very short time, in a few generations, we have gone from a relatively quiet natural electromagnetic environment to one that is literally packed with signals of every sort.

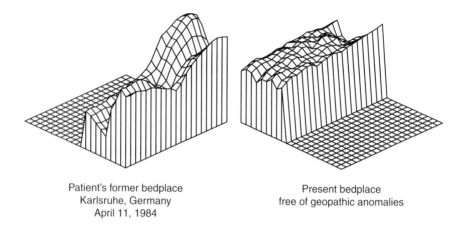

Patient's former bedplace
Karlsruhe, Germany
April 11, 1984

Present bedplace
free of geopathic anomalies

Fig. 13.5 Geopathic stress. Geopathic stress zones can be detected with a sensitive recording magnetometer that prints out a profile of the magnetic variations in an area such as a room or bedplace. Dowsing can also be used to detect these zones. Sometimes moving the bedplace from one side of a room to another, as shown here, reduces the geopathic stress on the occupant. Note the large peak or 'hot spot' in the former bedplace, and the relatively flat field profile after the bed was moved. Research cited here has shown that eliminating geopathic stress can have health benefits. (After Wooster 1988, with kind permission from the Townsend Letter for Doctors and Patients.)

Our technologies expose us to far more than a mixture of frequencies emitted by a host of devices. We enjoy a variety of appliances, such as electric blankets, hair dryers, food mixers, coffee mills, refrigerators, stoves, microwave ovens, sewing machines, coffee pots, heating pads, computers, televisions, radios, cell phones, water beds, etc. Each device produces a variety of signals while it is being used. Some of these energies are radiated directly into the tissues of nearby organisms, while some energy goes back into the power grid and travels a certain distance through it. Moreover, each device has controls that we use to turn it on and off, or to adjust its operations. Using each of these adjustments can set up transients, or pulses, or spikes with complex harmonics. These signals too are radiated into nearby tissues, and also enter the power distribution system and travel a certain distance. The pulses can interact with other fields and transients to produce complex interference patterns. These intricate and unpredictable signals can be conducted from one appliance to another, where they interact with another set of electrical or electronic components and the fields they are generating. Signals from radio, TV, cell phones, wireless pagers, satellite up-links and down-links, and natural geomagnetic and geoelectric phenomena can also be collected by the power

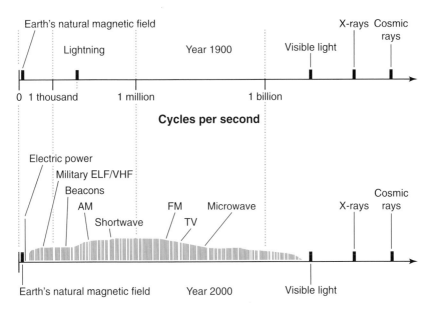

Fig. 13.6 The filling-in of the electromagnetic spectrum. During the last 100 years, our electromagnetic environment has gone from a naturally quiet place to one that is literally packed with signals of every sort. (After Becker 1990, pp 79,188,189, with kind permission from Robert O. Becker, MD.)

distribution grid, which acts as a huge antenna. All of these signals can interact to produce intense but unpredictable energetic 'hot spots' in particular regions of space.

'We have never encountered poor engineering in nature' (Albrecht-Buehler 1985). The electrical and electronic signals within the living system are honed to perfection. Each molecule has its electromagnetic signature (Oschman 1997b, Benveniste 1998). Each molecular interaction and each physiological process generates fields as well. All of these fields are compatible. In normal tissues, interferences and incompatibilities do not occur. Within the body, thousands of physiological and biochemical and electronic processes take place each second. Each heartbeat, each breath, each emotion generates characteristic electromagnetic fields that travel through the living matrix to cells and tissues a distance away. The result is coordination, integration, interdigitation of processes. When problems arise in this marvelous and intricate web, bodywork and movement therapies can restore order. In contrast to our organized and smoothly operating internal environment, the external electromagnetic background is chaotic and unpredictable.

Conclusions

Our present understanding of the natural and artificial energy fields in our environment is based on much careful research. This article provides a taste of the enormous amount of information that is available. The details are relevant to hands-on therapists of all schools who wish to educate themselves and their clients about both energy therapies and the invisible energies in their environment.

Three areas of investigation are particularly significant for developing a theoretical basis for energetic therapies of all kinds:

◆ Studies of the mechanisms by which sensory systems extract information from the environment

◆ Studies of the ways PEMF therapies trigger beneficial effects at the same frequencies and strengths as the signals emitted from the hands of therapists

◆ Studies of the tissue and cell effects of 50 and 60 cycle power signals, as well as microwaves and other radio frequencies.

The last of these will be discussed in the next chapter, which will also consider the potential hazards present in our electromagnetic environment and what can be done about them.

References

Adey W R 1980 Frequency and power windowing in tissue interactions with weak electromagnetic fields. Proceedings of the IEEE 68(1):119–125

Adey W R 1990 Electromagnetic fields and the essence of living systems: modern radio science. Oxford University Press, Oxford, pp 1–36

Adey W R, Bawin S M 1977 Brain interactions with weak electric and magnetic fields. Neurosciences Research Program Bulletin 15(1):1–129

Albrecht-Buehler G 1985 Is the cytoplasm intelligent too? Cell and Muscle Motility 6:1–21

Bassett C A L 1978 Pulsing electromagnetic fields: a new approach to surgical problems. In: Buchwald H, Varco R L (eds) Metabolic surgery. Grune & Stratton, NY, pp 255–306

Bassett C A L 1995 Bioelectromagnetics in the service of medicine. In: Blank M (ed) Electromagnetic fields: biological interactions and mechanisms. Advances in Chemistry Series 250. American Chemical Society, Washington DC, ch 14, pp 261–275

Bawin S M, Kaczmarek L K, Adey W R 1975 Effects of modulated very high frequency fields on specific brain rhythms in cats. Brain Research 58:365–384

Becker R O 1990 Cross currents: the perils of electropollution, the promise of electromedicine. Jeremy P. Tarcher, Los Angeles, CA

Bentor I 1976 Micromotion of the body as a factor in the development of the nervous system. In: Sannella L. Kundalini–Psychosis or Transcendence? H Dakin Co, San Francisco

Benveniste J 1998 From 'water memory effects' to 'digital biology.' On the web at: http://www.digibio.com/

Best S T 1988 What we don't know about earth radiation. Journal of Alternative and Complementary Medicine (November):17–18, 30

Bialek W 1987 Physical limits to sensation and perception. Annual Review of Biophysics and Biophysical Chemistry 16:455–478

Blackman C F, Elder J A, Weil C M, Benane S G, Eichinger D C, House D E 1979 Induction of calcium-ion efflux from brain tissue by radio-frequency radiation: effects of modulation frequency and field strength. Radio Science 14(6S):93–98

Bridges J E, Preache M 1981 Biological influences of power frequency electric fields: a tutorial review from a physical and experimental viewpoint. Proceedings of the IEEE 69(9):1092–1120

Chapman S, Bartels J 1940 Geomagnetism. Clarendon Press, Oxford

D'Arcy F J, Porter N A 1962 Detection of cosmic ray μ-mesons by the human eye. Nature 196(4858):1013–1014

Direnfeld L K 1983 The genesis of the EEG and its relation to electromagnetic radiation. Journal of Bioelectricity 2:111–121

Dubrov A P 1978 The geomagnetic field and life: geomagnetobiology. Plenum Press, New York

Foster K R, Guy A W 1986 The microwave problem. Scientific American 255(3):32–39

Foster K R, Pickard W F 1987 Microwaves: the risks of risk research. Nature 330:531–532

Fröhlich H 1968a Bose condensation of strongly excited longitudinal electric modes. Physics Letters 26A:402–403

Fröhlich H 1968b Long-range coherence and energy storage in biological systems. International Journal of Quantum Chemistry 2:641–649

Fröhlich H 1970 Long-range coherence and the action of enzymes. Nature 228:1093

Fröhlich H 1974 Possibilities of long- and short-range electric interactions of biological systems. In: Adey W R, Bawin S M (eds) Brain interactions with weak electric and magnetic fields. Neurosciences Research Program Bulletin 15:1–129

Fröhlich H 1975 Evidence for bose condensation-like excitation of coherent modes in biological systems. Physics Letters 51A:21–22

Fröhlich H (ed) 1988 Biological coherence and response to external stimuli. Springer-Verlag, Berlin

Gordon R 1988 Are you sleeping in a safe place? Dulwich Health Society, London

Graham G 1724 An account of observations made of the variation of the horizontal needle at London, in the latter part of the year 1722. Philosophical Transactions of the Royal Society of London, Series A, 32:96–107

Guy A W, Chou C K, Lin J C, Christensen D 1975 Microwave induced acoustic effects in mammalian auditory systems and physical materials. Annals of the New York Academy of Sciences 247:194–218

Hansteen C 1819 Untersuchungen über den Magnetismus der Erde. Lehmann & Gröndahl, Christiania

Ho M-W 1998 The rainbow and the worm: the physics of organisms, 2nd edn. World Scientific, River Edge, NJ

Ho M-W, Popp F-A, Warnke U 1994 Bioelectrodynamics and biocommunication. World Scientific, Singapore

Hoyle F 1962 Astronomy. Crescent Books, Inc.

Jacobs J A (ed) 1987 Geomagnetism. 4 vols. Academic Press, London

Kalmijn A J 1971 The electric sense of sharks and rays. Journal of Experimental Biology 55(2):371–383

Lednev V V 1991 Possible mechanism for the influence of weak magnetic fields on biological systems. Bioelectromagnetics 12(2):71–75

Liboff A R 1985 Cyclotron resonance in membrane transport. In: Chiabrera A, Nicolini C, Schwan H P (eds) Interactions between electromagnetic fields and cells. Plenum Press, New York, pp 281–296

Malin S 1987. Historical introduction to geomagnetism. In: Jacobs J A (ed) Geomagnetism. Academic Press, London, vol 1, ch 1, pp 1–49

Matsushita S, Campbell W H (eds) 1967 Physics of geomagnetic phenomena. Academic Press, New York

Miller A 1998 Dowsing: a review. Network 66:3–8

Murchie G 1978 The seven mysteries of life. Houghton Mifflin, Boston

Oschman J L 1997a Healing energy, part 3: silent pulses. Journal of Bodywork and Movement Therapies 1(3):179–194

Oschman J L 1997b Healing energy, part 4: vibrational medicines. Journal of Bodywork and Movement Therapies 1(4):239–250

Oschman J L (2000) Energy medicine: the new paradigm. In: Charman R (ed) Complementary therapies for physical therapists: theoretical and clinical exploration. Butterworth Heinemann, Oxford, introductory chapter

Presman AS 1970 Electromagnetic fields and life. Plenum Press, New York.

Schienle A, Stark R, Vaitl D 1998 Biological effects of very low frequency (VLF) atmospherics in humans: a review. Journal of Scientific Exploration 12(3):455–468

Schumann WO König H 1954 Über die Beobachtung von Atmospheics bei geringstein Frequenzen. Naturwissenschaften 41:183

Sentman DD 1995 Schumann resonances. In: Volland H (ed) Handbook of atmospheric electrodynamics. CRC Press, Boca Raton, vol 1, pp 267–295

Smith CW, Best S 1989 Electromagnetic man: health and hazard in the electrical environment. Dent, London.

Stryer L 1985 Molecular design of an amplification cascade in vision. Biopolymers 24(1): 29–47

Stryer L 1987 The molecules of visual excitation. Scientific American 257(1): 42–50

Stryer L 1988 Molecular basis of visual excitation. Cold Spring Harbor

Symposium on Quantitative Biology 52:283–294

Valet J-P, Meynadier L 1993 Geomagnetic field intensity and reversals during the past four million years. Nature 366 (6452): 234–238

Volland H 1984 Handbook of atmospheric electrodynamics. CRC Press, Boca Raton.

von Aschoff D 1986 Geopathische Zonen-physikalische Grundlage der Krebsentstehung. Presented at the International Congress ZDN, Essen, 19 October 1985. Mehr Wisen Buch-Deinst, Dusseldorf

von Pohl GF 1985 Earth currents: Causative factor of cancer and other diseases. Translation of 1932 original by I Lang, Frech-Verlag, Stuttgart.

Wachtel H 1995 Comparison of endogenous currents in and around cells with those induced by exogenous extremely low frequency magnetic fields. In: Blank M (ed) Electromagnetic fields: biological interactions and mechanisms. Advances in Chemistry Series 250. American Chemical Society, Washington DC, ch 6, pp 99–107

Warnke U 1994 Electromagnetic sensitivity of animals and humans: biological and clinical implications. In: Ho M-W, Popp F-A, Warnke U (eds) Bioelectrodynamics and biocommunication. World Scientific, Singapore, ch 15, p 365–386

Wienert KA 1970 Notes on geomagnetic observatory and survey practice. UNESCO, Paris

Wick GL 1972 Cosmic rays: detection with the eye. Science 175:615–616

Wooster S M 1988 Geopathogenic stress and cancer. Townsend Letter for Doctors and Patients 64:482–483

14 The electromagnetic environment: biological effects

Introduction

The question of all questions for humanity, the problem which lies behind all others and is more interesting than any of them, is that of the determination of [our] place in nature and [our] relation to the cosmos.
(T. H. Huxley, quoted in Seymour 1988, p. 211)

About 2500 years ago, Hippocrates recognized the significance of the weather and climate on living systems (Jones 1948). In the 20th century, the relations between natural electromagnetic rhythms and living systems were explored in the pioneering work of Harold Saxton Burr and his colleagues at Yale University School of Medicine (for references see Burr 1957). In the 1950s, a visitor to Burr's ancestral home, Mansewood, in Lyme, Connecticut, would discover various kinds of trees connected to recording voltmeters. Burr was studying how the electric fields of trees change in advance of weather patterns and other atmospheric phenomena. His research had convinced him that life on earth is not isolated from the rest of the universe, but is susceptible to forces extending across vast distances of space. The fields within the human body are inevitably affected by the larger fields of the planet and other celestial bodies. The mechanisms involved are not mystical or obscure – they involve well-documented pathways of interaction. For example, sunspots and the cycles of the moon cause changes in ionospheric currents and geophysical fields which in turn influence the fields within us.

To Burr it was obvious that the energies so thoroughly studied by physicists surround, penetrate, and are produced by every organism. He was convinced that all living things, from mice to men, from seeds to trees, are formed and controlled by fields that can be measured with standard detectors. The fields reflect physical and mental conditions, and can therefore be useful for diagnosis. Burr obtained evidence that abnormal fields show up before serious pathology sets in, and that balancing or restoring the field can reverse disease processes.

These concepts are also part of the core theory of acupuncture and related methods, and are being validated by modern biomedical research on cancer and AIDS (Brewitt 1996, 1999).

Burr's discoveries paralleled those of another controversial scientist, Frank A. Brown, Jr., who documented the abilities of plants and animals to synchronize their biological clocks with the large-scale rhythms of nature (Brown 1973). In addition to a lifetime of research on biological clocks, Brown was responsible for the translations into English of two valuable books, *Electromagnetic Fields and Life* (Presman 1970) and *The Geomagnetic Field and Life* (Dubrov 1978).

Another important investigator in this area was Gauguelin (1966, 1974). The conclusions of all of these scientists regarding the externally driven biological clocks were confirmed by Wever (1968), who showed that shielding humans from natural electromagnetic fields desynchronized their biological rhythms. Further confirmation came from studies of the relations between reaction time and ELF micropulsations from approaching thunderstorms (Reiter 1953, Moore-Ede et al 1992).

All of the scientists mentioned above were following in the footsteps of one of the world's foremost chemists, Svante Arrhenius, who developed the theory for the way salts dissolve in water, and then went on to study the relationships between environmental fields and health (see Ward 1971). Arrhenius's profound insight came in a flash on the night of May 17, 1883. After a sleepless night, working through the concept, Arrhenius raced to his thesis advisor to present his theory. His professor looked at him through skeptical eyes and said, 'You have a new theory? That is very interesting. Goodbye'.

Arrhenius's doctoral thesis was graded 'fourth class' by the then conservative faculty at the University of Uppsala. His ideas challenged concepts of the establishment, and were strongly opposed. It was years before his theory came to be accepted by chemists everywhere, leading to great progress. In 1903, Arrhenius received the Nobel Prize, and in 1909, King Oscar II installed him as director of the Nobel Institute for Physical Chemistry at Stockholm. Here Arrhenius was given the situation every scientist dreams of: ideal conditions to study whatever interested him.

Soon Arrhenius turned his attention to cosmic influences on the behavior of plants, animals, and humans. He found data on the periodic occurrence of bronchitis, epilepsy, birth and death rates, and the human ovulation cycle. He concluded that biological rhythms correlate with rhythms and tides in the cosmic forces that surround the earth. He suggested that the electrical tension in the air influences biochemical reactions and thereby affects all living things. His work laid the groundwork for one of the stormiest controversies of modern biology.

Weather sensitivity

A large percentage of the population is weather sensitive (reviewed by Schienle et al 1998). Those who are unaware of this phenomenon are puzzled by the sudden onset of headaches, sleepiness, indigestion, phantom limb pain, asthma, sleep disorders, fatigue, confusion, or other symptoms, often prior to weather changes. Part of the problem is that a lightning storm can precipitate physiological changes, and then swerve off in a different direction, leaving the weather-sensitive individual unaware of the cause of discomfort. Emotional and behavioral changes and their consequences have also been observed: increases in crime rates, suicides, memory loss, lack of concentration, prolonged reaction times, and automobile and industrial accidents.

Allergies

Information about environmental electromagnetic fields is of increasing importance as more and more people are developing electromagnetic sensitivities (Smith & Best 1989; Best 1984, 1988; Choy et al 1987). The father of electrical engineering, Nikolai Tesla, was probably the first well-documented but non-diagnosed case of electromagnetic hypersensitivity (Smith & Best 1989). Some individuals are, in essence, allergic to 50 or 60 Hz electromagnetic fields. These are people who immediately react when they are near transformers, fluorescent lights, microwave ovens, refrigerators, and other appliances. Often these are multiple allergy patients.

Multiple sensitivity begins when a person is exposed to a chemical agent, such as a pesticide, drug, solvent, perfume, smoke, exhaust, or chemicals in food or in carpets. The agent (or its electromagnetic signature – see below) triggers a reaction in one or more of the body's regulatory systems. The result of the initial encounter can be fatigue, respiratory problems, or difficulty concentrating. After one is sensitized, future exposures to even minute amounts of the allergen can trigger an immediate reaction. The problem is compounded when the sensitized person is exposed to a second agent, or to an electromagnetic field, while reacting to the first allergen. In this way, people can develop allergies to hundreds of substances and their electromagnetic signatures. Few physicians understand electromagnetic sensitivities, and therefore treat the symptoms without recognizing the source of the problem.

To treat electromagnetic allergies, Smith and colleagues use a clinical confrontation-neutralization protocol. The principle is the same as that used in the classical skin tests for chemical allergies. A signal generator a distance from the patient is used to find the frequency that will trigger the allergic reaction. Then other frequencies are tested to find the neutralizing frequencies that stop the reaction. Signals at these frequencies can 'potentize' vials of water that can be carried by the patient and used to stop the reaction. The allergic response is inhibited by holding the vial of water in the hand. In a given patient, the symptoms provoked electrically are similar to those provoked chemically and those provoked by the patient's environment. Electrical and chemical stimuli and neutralization appear to be interchangeable (Choy et al 1987, Smith & Best 1989).

'Billiard ball' regulations vs electromagnetic signaling

The research of Smith (1987) and Benveniste (1998), and others cited below, provides dramatic documentation of an important phenomenon that underlies a number of energetic therapies as well as environmental electromagnetic effects.

In the conventional picture of biological regulations (left side of Fig. 14.1) structurally matching molecules exchange energy and information by billiard-ball type direct impacts. Signal molecules diffuse, wiggle, and bump about randomly until they chance to approach a receptor site, at which time electrostatic, short-range (two to three times the molecule size) forces draw them together so that 'the key can fit into the lock'. It is not generally appreciated that this kind of random encounter, taking place in a sea of other molecules, gives these molecular meetings a statistically low probability. The simplest biological event or regulatory process should require a very long time to happen.

In the energetic model of biological regulations (shown to the right in Fig. 14.1), communication occurs between signal and receptor molecules that are not touching (Benveniste 1998). The term 'molecular signal' acquires an electromagnetic meaning. In essence, the molecules interact by coresonance, like radio transmitters and receivers. If you tune a receiver to 92.6 MHz, you tune in Station A, because electrons in the antennas of the receiver and the transmitter are oscillating at the same frequency. If you tune the receiver to a different frequency, say 91.6 MHz, you receive Station B instead. In living systems, long-range electromagnetic fields transmit messages between distant molecules, as long as their emission and absorption spectra match. Non-resonating, unwanted random signals are excluded. From basic electronics, we know that particularly good reception – meaning good separation of signal from noise – takes place if the transmitting and receiving antennas have the same length and orientation.

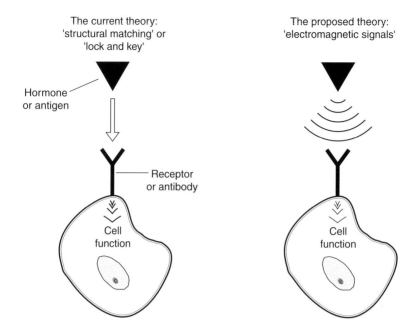

Fig. 14.1 Theories of molecular signaling. To the left, the conventional structural matching or 'lock and key' model of biological regulations. The three-dimensional structure of a ligand molecule, such as a hormone, antigen, or other signal molecule matches the three-dimensional structure of the receptor or antibody. This physical contact activates a particular cell function. To the right is the proposed electromagnetic model. The signal molecule emits an electromagnetic signal (signature) which coresonates with the receptor molecule, thereby activating it and triggering the cell function. (After Benveniste 1998, with kind permission from Dr J. Benveniste.)

Molecular electromagnetic communications can account for the rapid and subtle and integrated functioning of living systems. Millions of molecules can communicate with each other in this way. The upper limit on the signal velocity is the speed of light.

Dramatic evidence for this electromagnetic resonance model comes from studies of molecular signals recorded and digitized with a multimedia computer sound card (Benveniste 1998). A molecular signal is represented by a spectrum of frequencies in the range 20–20000 Hz, similar to the range of human hearing and music. In thousands of experiments, repeated over many years, Benveniste has shown that playing recordings of the electromagnetic signatures of signal molecules can trigger various kinds of receptors to respond, just as though they were in the presence of the molecules that normally trigger them.

The mechanisms behind molecular coresonance are well understood. We have known for over a century that atoms and molecules vibrate when they absorb or emit electromagnetic waves. The resulting electromagnetic 'signatures' are used by spectroscopists to determine molecular structure and to identify unknown molecules. Most of what we know about the molecular structure of drugs and antibiotics comes from spectroscopic data. And, radio telescopes detect characteristic molecular signals at distances of billions of light-years.

From the research of Smith (1987) and Benveniste (1998), and their colleagues, there is every reason to think that signal molecules can activate their corresponding receptor sites without physical contact. The signal molecule emits frequencies that resonate with the receptor and cause it to vibrate as well. For example, when you are in a dangerous situation, adrenalin 'tells' its various receptors, and those receptors alone, to make your heart beat faster, to dilate pupils and superficial blood vessels, and to trigger the other reactions of the 'fight or flight' response. Benveniste has suggested that the specific actions of biomolecules (e.g. histamine, caffeine, nicotine, adrenalin, insulin, etc.), as well as the antigens of viruses and bacteria, are due more to electromagnetic interactions than to direct contact.

These findings have enormous therapeutic implications and provide new insights into the energetic interactions taking place between and within organisms. They also provide clues about how environmental fields can influence physiological processes.

The legacy of Lucretian biochemistry

Smith (1987) and Benveniste (1998) are among the minority of scientists who have considered the possibility that electromagnetic signaling can play a direct communication role in living matter. Albert Szent-Györgyi was another. In the following quotation he refers to the biochemistry based on the ancient concepts of Lucretius and Epicurus, who pioneered the idea that matter is composed of hard, indivisible 'billiard-ball' units, atoms:

> Lucretian biochemistry involves the assumption that no interaction can take place between molecules without their touching one another. Support is given in this book [Szent-Györgyi 1957] to the idea that manifold interactions can take place without such bodily contact, either through energy bands or through the electromagnetic field, which thus appears with water and its structures as the matrix of biological reactions. Water does not merely fill the space between molecules. Water is more than this; it is part and parcel of the living matter itself. One of the main functions of the protoplasmic structures

[cytoskeleton and nuclear matrix] may be to generate in water those specific structures which make forms of electronic excitations and energy transmissions possible which would be improbable outside these structures. (Szent-Györgyi 1957) [statements in brackets added]

The importance of water cannot be overemphasized. In terms of electronics, the essential role of water structure Szent-Györgyi referred to is impedance matching between the oscillating molecule and the propagating medium. Impedance matching is essential for efficient transmission of energy. Stated another way, water both conditions and is conditioned by the molecular framework in cells and tissues, the living matrix.

In spite of all of the documentation and its conceptual simplicity, electromagnetic interactions have been difficult for many scientists to grasp. This is remarkable, considering that action at a distance is an accepted part of Newtonian mechanics, and accounts for the motions of the celestial bodies. Newtonian mechanics justifies movements other than those produced by impulsion.

None of the work on electromagnetic interactions between molecules violates any of the known laws of chemistry, physics, or biology. The passage from a biology of rigid structures randomly bumping into each other to one of information traveling at the speed of light can be accomplished without a 'scientific revolution'. All of the pieces of the puzzle are well accepted.

Acute pathology

Geomagnetic storms often begin with turmoil on the sun. The sun spews very fast and energetic blobs of matter and magnetic energy that are carried earthward by the solar wind. When this energy crashes into the earth's magnetosphere, enormous electrical currents are set up. These currents, in turn, influence the huge electric currents flowing in the ionosphere. Geomagnetic storms can be so intense that they damage satellites, power lines, telephone cables, and pipelines, and disrupt radio communications. It is not surprising that these events, which can be intense enough to prevent your automobile from starting, can affect physiology and behavior. Geomagnetic disturbances have been correlated with the onset of a variety of disorders and death. The following list includes a sample of the enormous literature on this subject:

◆ Cardiovascular problems (Bellossi et al 1985; Watanabe et al 1994; Stoupel et al 1993, 1994, 1995; Knox et al 1979)

◆ Seizures, epilepsy, convulsions (Stoupel et al 1991, Mikulecky et al 1996, Persinger & Psych 1995)

- ◆ Hypothermia (Bureau et al 1996)

- ◆ Headache (De Matteis et al 1994)

- ◆ Vestibular problems (Persinger & Richards 1995)

- ◆ Bacterial growth (Polikarpov 1996)

- ◆ Intraocular pressure (Stoupel et al 1993)

- ◆ Sleep (Kotleba et al 1973, Conesa 1995)

- ◆ Death (Lipa et al 1976, Stocks 1925).

In addition, a variety of behavioral changes have been noted:

- ◆ Crime (Chibrikin et al 1995)

- ◆ Aggression (St Pierre & Persinger 1998)

- ◆ Anxiety (Usenko & Panin 1993)

- ◆ Depression (Kay 1994)

- ◆ Loss of attention and memory (Tambiev et al 1995)

- ◆ Accidents (Grigor'ev 1995).

Efforts to replicate these studies have yielded conflicting results. The reasons such studies are difficult to reproduce have been discussed in detail by Hainsworth (1983). The main problem is that living systems are exquisitely sensitive to low energy signals, and individuals vary widely in their responses. Some individuals are affected negatively, some are neutral, and others seem to benefit from geomagnetic storms and related meteorological phenomena. Because of this, massive amounts of data are needed to establish valid relationships. (See section on scalar waves below, for a perspective on individual variation that relates to structural bodywork.)

To complement the correlation studies, some researchers have simulated geomagnetic variations to induce seizures (e.g. Michon et al 1996, Michon & Persinger 1997, Persinger 1996, Schienle et al 1998), changes in reaction time (Reiter 1953), and other effects.

Reviews of earlier literature have been published by Rajaram & Mitra (1981) and Venkataraman (1976). The latter author suggests that the effects of pulsing magnetic fields are similar to the well-known photoflash phenomenon that induces seizures. This is a reasonable hypothesis, given that virtually any form of pulsating energy can entrain brain waves (see Oschman 1997, Di Perri 1972, Alexander & Gray 1972, Foster 1975).

Electromagnetic pollution and other diseases

While there is heated debate, many serious health problems, including cancer, are being correlated with exposure to the invisible electromagnetic radiation produced by 50 and 60 cycle appliances, microwaves, radio transmitters, computers, etc. (some of the literature on this subject is listed in Appendix II). Serious problems have also been correlated with 'geopathic stress' (see Ch. 13).

Chapter 13 described the great sensitivity organisms have to exceedingly tiny signals in their environment, and the reasons many physicists reached the conclusion that the biology was simply wrong. This physics/biology dilemma was resolved in the late 1970s when it became clear that the living systems completely defy the logic that larger stimuli should produce larger responses. Living tissues are non-linear, cooperative, and coherent, and are capable of responding to very specific 'windows' in terms of frequency and intensity (Fig. 13.1). Thus information on the health effects of natural and artificial electromagnetic fields is understandable on the basis of what has been learned about the sensitivities of all living systems to minute environmental signals. Interference with the molecular electromagnetic regulatory systems depicted in Figure 14.1 undoubtedly also play a role.

The previous chapter also mentioned the Fröhlich model, in which the sensitivity of living systems is accounted for on the basis of the large numbers of molecules that form regular arrays, similar to those found in radio telescope antennas. Teneforde & Kaune (1987) list a number of other models that are under consideration. In any case, electromagnetic fields in the extremely low frequency range (which includes the 50 and 60 power distribution system) now have well-documented effects on a wide range of cellular systems.

R.P. Liburdy and colleages have studied the effects of electromagnetic fields on cultured cells. Under well-controlled conditions, they established unequivocal field effects and identified the sites of action in the cellular regulatory process. However, a Federal Ethics Inquiry has recently found Liburdy guilty of 'scientific misconduct'. Supposedly he falsified and fabricated data published in two papers published in 1992.

After discussions with experts in the field, I suspect Liburdy was treated unfairly by the engineering of absurd and irrelevant statements prominently reported in the media. On page 1 of the New York Times (July 24, 1999) we find: 'The disclosure [of Liburdy's 'misconduct'] appears to strengthen the case that electric power is safe'. In the Wall Street Journal (July 27, 1999, p. A22): 'A government-funded scientist systematically distorted data to support the hypothesis that electromagnetic fields near powerlines cause cancer'. And, in Science (July 2, 1999): 'EMF researcher made up data'. These preposterous headlines have virtually nothing to do with Liburdy and his research. Liburdy never stated that, 'electromagnetic fields near powerlines cause cancer'. Actually, his data and interpretations were not challenged in the ethics review, just how the data were graphed. Moreover, Liburdy is widely respected, and his key conclusions have been confirmed in other laboratories. Here are some of the findings:

◆ Radiofrequency radiation affects the immune system by altering human immunoglobulin on T- and B-lymphocytes. The effect takes place at power levels below the current USA recommended safety limit of 0.4 W kg^{-1} (Liburdy & Wyant 1984).

◆ Microwaves at 2450 MHz increase the sodium permeability of rabbit erythrocytes (Liburdy & Vanek 1985) and cause the shedding of at least 11 proteins from the cell surface (Liburdy et al 1988).

◆ The calcium channel is the site of field interactions (Liburdy 1992).

◆ The findings on calcium metabolism are consistent with a proposed parametric resonance theory of the interaction of low intensity magnetic fields with biological systems (Lednev 1991, Yost & Liburdy 1992).

◆ 60 Hz magnetic fields enhance breast cancer cell proliferation by blocking melatonin's natural oncostatic action. The effect is 'windowed' between 2 and 12 mG (milli Gauss) (Liburdy et al 1993a).

◆ Magnetic fields, mitogens and carcinogens influence the cascade of regulatory signal transduction processes. An early effect is on calcium influx into the cell, followed by an effect on the expression of a specific gene. A very weak dose of a mitogen, insufficient to trigger cell proliferation by itself, will stimulate cell division if it is combined with 60 Hz field treatment (Liburdy et al 1993b).

◆ Both melatonin and tamoxifen inhibit the growth of cultured human breast cancer cells. 60 Hz fields block these inhibitions (Harland & Liburdy 1997).

Statements by physicists such as Bennett (1994) that the fields from appliances cannot possibly affect living systems, are simply outdated. Much more up-to-date information can be found in a wide variety of scientific journals, in a bi-annual series entitled *Advances in Electromagnetic Fields in Living Systems* (Lin 1994, 1997), and has been the subject of at least two Congressional hearings.

The relevance to the energy therapist is that the studies are showing that electromagnetic fields, at the frequencies and intensities emitted from the hands of a therapist, are capable of producing biological effects. It appears that the low frequencies emitted from the hands of therapists, and from pulsing electromagnetic field therapy devices (in the range of 2-30 Hz) are beneficial, whereas somewhat higher frequencies of the power distribution system (50 and 60 Hz) are harmful.

Scalar waves

Physics has a little-known framework for a deeper understanding of electric and magnetic fields and their biological effects. Research in this area has considerable therapeutic significance. The concepts involved go to the heart of the quantum mechanical interpretation of reality and consciousness.

Briefly, we learn in classical physics that waves can interfere with each other. When two waves are of the same frequency and are *in phase* (the timing of their variations is identical), their amplitudes add together to create larger waves (Fig. 14.2A–C). This is termed *constructive* interference. When the waves are exactly *out of phase*, their amplitudes subtract, and they can partially or completely cancel or destroy each other. This is termed *destructive* interference (Fig. 14.2D–F). In nature, interacting waves usually have a mix of frequencies and phases, and therefore add and subtract in a complex manner.

The field concept originated with Michael Faraday in 1846. However, the introduction of relativity and quantum mechanics shortly after the beginning of the 20th century required that fields be expressed in terms of a more fundamental entity, called potentials. Whittaker (1903, 1904) recognized this, and Tesla (1904) generated potential waves and called them 'non-Hertzian waves'. When we say that a magnetic field induces a current flow in a conductor, such as a wire or a living tissue, it is actually the potential component of the field, and not the field itself, that underlies the effect. The potentials are of two kinds, called electric scalar potentials and magnetic vector potentials.

For a long time, it was thought that these potentials had no real existence or significance. They were created as abstractions that were needed to simplify and balance quantum equations. That there was far more to the story was

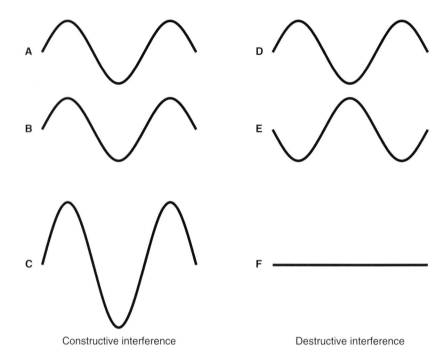

Constructive interference   Destructive interference

Fig. 14.2 Interference. In constructive interference **(A,B,C)** waves that are in phase add together to produce a larger wave. In destructive interference **(D,E,F)** waves that are out of phase with each other can cancel or destroy each other.

revealed in a classic paper by Aharonov & Bohm (1959). These authors showed that the potentials must have a physical reality, and suggested some experiments to demonstrate them.

The first demonstration of a magnetic vector potential was done with a coil designed so that the electric and magnetic fields remained entirely within its core, and absolutely no field existed on the outside. A beam of electrons passing through the 'force-free' region around the coil nonetheless underwent a phase change, indicating that some non-electric, non-magnetic physical 'entity' must be acting on it. This entity is the magnetic vector potential.

Subsequent work documented the existence of an electric scalar potential in a region where no electric field exists. Both of these phenomena are referred to as the Aharonov–Bohm effect, a cornerstone of quantum mechanics. Technical details were published by Olariu & Popescu (1985). (For a less technical but still challenging account, see Imry & Webb 1989.)

Hence, in destructive interference, where the classical fields cancel each other, there nonetheless remain electrostatic scalar potentials and magnetic vector potentials. In essence, the energy and information contained in the original waves is not *destroyed* by interference. In fact, the classical electromagnetic field is actually derived from two potential waves interfering with each other.

The Aharonov–Bohm effect began as an abstraction needed to balance quantum equations, but gradually found its way into down-to-earth applications in electronics. Scalar waves have been utilized for a communication system (Gelinas 1984) and for a device for locating humans and other animals during rescue-search operations (Afilani 1998).

Various kinds of coil designs enable the vectors (the directions and magnitudes) of the electric and magnetic fields to destructively interfere or cancel each other (Fig. 14.3). The Figure legend describes the kinds of waves and fields they produce.

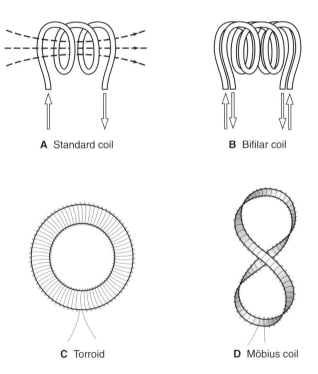

A Standard coil   **B** Bifilar coil

C Torroid   **D** Möbius coil

Fig. 14.3 Coils used to emit fields and potentials. **A** A standard coil emits electric and magnetic fields in the space around it. **B** In the bifilar coil the electric and magnetic fields are canceled, and electric scalar and magnetic vector waves are produced. **C** The torroidal coil has the same effect. **D** The Möbius coil produces only scalar waves. The information on coil properties is from Abraham (1998).

Scalar waves appear to interact with atomic nuclei, rather than with electrons. Such interactions are described by quantum chromodynamics (Ynduráin 1983). The waves are not blocked by Faraday cages or other kinds of shielding, they are probably emitted by living systems, and they appear to be intimately involved in healing (see e.g. Jacobs 1997, Rein 1998).

The scalar potential has a peculiarity: it propagates instantaneously everywhere in space, undiminished by distance. In contrast, the vector potential has a finite velocity (Jackson 1975). In the real world, scalar waves encounter environmental fields, and complex interactions take place that prevent them from extending indefinitely into space. Mathematical physics justifies the instantaneous propagation of scalar waves, but this is often dismissed as 'obviously unphysical behavior' (e.g. Jackson 1975).

The present situation parallels what happened over a century ago with regard to electromagnetic fields. When Maxwell combined the understandings that had been reached by Faraday, Ampère, and Gauss, he declared that there must exist an 'electromagnetic wave' capable of transmitting energy at a speed of 300 million m/sec. At the time, the suggestion was considered to be completely outrageous. Subsequently, Hertz showed that Maxwell was correct, and Marconi applied the phenomenon when he developed practical radio transmission. Many times in our history, the mathematics requires a phenomenon to exist, but it takes years to demonstrate it.

Much more is known about electric and magnetic fields than about scalar waves and vector potentials, simply because fields are easy to measure. Experimental demonstration of scalar waves and vector potentials, and their biological effects, is extremely difficult. At present, the best way to document their presence is by testing on electromagnetically sensitive individuals. It is widely assumed that it is the electric and magnetic fields that interact with organisms, but some researchers suspect that scalar and potential waves actually underlie these effects.

Scalar waves and bodywork

For the evolution of energetic bodywork and energy medicine, a number of important consequences are emerging from research on scalar waves. Each bioelectric and biomagnetic field produced by the human body – whether emitted by the brain, the heart, the eye, the muscles, an organ, or by the hand of a therapist, or a QiGong practitioner – will also be associated with scalar waves and vector potentials.

It is important to look at the ways in which the energetic anatomy of the body might give rise to self-canceling fields that result in biological scalar waves. Moreover, the energy fields in the environment, whether natural or created by technology, also have scalar and vector components. For example, the Schumann resonance (see Chs 7 and 13) is described by five quantities: velocity of propagation, electric field, magnetic field, electric scalar potential, and magnetic vector potential (Abraham, personal communication 1998). Further research is needed to determine the extent to which the biological effects of the Schumann resonance, VLF-sferics, and geopathic stress, as well as the phenomenon of dowsing, are related to the Aharonov–Bohm effect.

Near field interactions occur when the interacting elements, such as a therapist and patient, are close enough that their energy fields, which abruptly drop off in strength with distance, can interact. What about other healing modalities that seem independent of distance? A large and growing body of reliable evidence shows that intercessory prayer is effective, even when the patients and those praying for them are separated by great distances (Dossey 1993).

The idea of subtle interactions at a distance is embodied in the 'synchronicity' concept of Jung (Peat 1987), and is also part of radionics and related methods (e.g. Fellows 1997). While these and kindred phenomena, such as telepathy and clairvoyance, are too far-fetched for some scientists, there is now too much evidence to ignore them (see a thorough discussion in Woodhouse 1996).

Some scholars look to the well-documented peculiarities of quantum mechanics for explanations, such as quantum non-locality (Rohrlich 1983). It is often stated that non-local phenomena are mediated by unknown forms of energy, sometimes vaguely referred to as 'subtle energies'. Some look to these phenomena for clues about the nature of consciousness and the structure of the physical universe. Others suggest the word 'energy' is inadequate, and its use in relation to healing should be discontinued. The philosophical and metaphysical implications are the subject of ongoing discussions (e.g. exchanges between Dossey and Woodhouse in Network 64, 1997).

Key studies of non-local interactions have been published by Grinberg-Zylberbaum and colleagues (1992, 1994). Pairs of subjects who achieve a feeling of emotional connection (empathy) can develop correlated electroencephalographic (EEG) patterns that are not attenuated by spatial separation or by electromagnetic shielding (Faraday cages). When one of the subjects was stimulated, as with a flash of light, the evoked brainwave was 'transferred' to a non-stimulated subject in another electromagnetically shielded room. The researchers assert that these findings represent a genuinely non-local, macroscopic manifestation of consciousness that is physiologically relevant.

Studies like this, using shielded rooms, seem to rule out energetic interactions; but do they? What about the scalar and vector potentials described above. Could the Aharonov–Bohm effect account for non-local interactions?

One possibility is that long-range biological interactions may be due to modulation of the scalar component of the Schumann resonance (Oschman 2000). While this may seem far-fetched, it is fascinating that well-documented 'telepathic experiences' are reliably and systematically correlated with calm periods of global geomagnetic activity (Persinger & Krippner 1993).

Implications for structural bodywork

Ida Rolf emphasized the importance of the relationship between fields of the living body and the larger fields of the planet (Rolf 1962). As deep tissue alignment methods (e.g. Rolfing®, structural integration, etc.) and related techniques bring the body into anatomical and energetic balance with the field of gravity, it is possible that conditions may also develop such that the bioelectric and/or biomagnetic fields partly cancel each other. In such circumstances, the measured biomagnetic field would be converted into scalar and/or vector potentials. How this would affect an individual can only be a fascinating speculation at the present time. One possibility is that an individual capable of generating significant scalar waves would be relatively protected from negative effects of environmental energies. Perhaps this can explain the phenomenon mentioned above, that there is a wide range in responses in weather sensitive people. While some individuals suffer, others seem to enjoy the stimulatory effects of geomagnetic storms and related meteorological events.

Prudent avoidance

In the 1980s, several personal electromagnetic shielding devices were developed – based on the use of coils of the Möbius design that emit scalar waves – which were said to be safe for living systems. One of these devices was a watch containing a microchip that produced a Schumann-type signal at about 8.0 Hz. This device purportedly stabilized a person's brain waves at a frequency that was considered safe and beneficial. Many of these devices were sold, and there were reports of benefits from wearing them, including reduction of jet lag, more energy, lower blood pressure, feelings of well-being, etc. These qualitative effects have been difficult to document.

Rein (1998) has summarized more recent work on the biological effects of scalar waves. Scalar waves can inhibit neurotransmitter uptake into nerve cells and stimulate the growth of human lymphocytes. There are indications that the effects are in part mediated by effects on the properties of cell and tissue water.

Recently, more powerful emitters of scalar waves, in the range 6–60 milliwatts power consumption, have been developed (Abraham 1998). The devices emit scalar waves at the average Schumann frequency, 7.83 Hz. Preliminary tests indicate that scalar waves at this frequency are safe, and protect those who suffer from electromagnetic field sensitivity. Moreover, clinical trials in progress are indicating a variety of health benefits, including improvement of symptoms of chronic fatigue syndrome, fibromyalgia, cognitive impairments, and sleep disorders (Abraham, personal communication 1998).

The development of a reliable and powerful source of potential waves opens up many possibilities for studies of the clinical effects of this form of energy, and, possibly, for resolving some of the mysteries and variability of both local and non-local biological effects.

There is widespread confusion and misinformation about our electromagnetic environment. Key information widely available in technical circles is virtually unknown to the general public. This is due to several factors that reinforce each other. One is the strong bias many biologists have against geophysical pacemakers for biological rhythms. This bias arises in part because evidence of this sort might be taken as support for astrology, a subject that is widely considered to be scientifically unfounded (see, however, Seymour 1988). Another is the threat to the ego posed by the possibility that our lives might be influenced by events very far away from us. The idea that the human body both radiates and is sensitive to invisible energy fields may be menacing to some. Finally, a documentation of health effects from fields generated by power distribution systems and technological devices have enormous economic and legal consequences.

Therapists are careful to make their treatment spaces as pleasant and comfortable as possible. But what about the ubiquitous invisible energies present in the treatment environment? No matter how well you treat individuals with electromagnetic or geopathic sensitivities and related disorders, they will continue to have problems when they go back to their homes and/or workplaces where they are immersed in disturbing energy fields. Treating the whole person involves education about the possible health effects of the invisible electromagnetic environment so that suitable precautions can be taken.

These considerations are of increasing importance for a variety of reasons that have been discussed here. Moreover, the likely physiological effects of environmental fields have been more widely researched than many people realize. Virtually every disease and disorder has been linked by one investigator or another to electromagnetic pollution. As one example, Sobel and colleagues have noted an elevated risk of Alzheimer's disease among those who work in areas where they are exposed to high electromagnetic fields (Sobel et al 1995a, 1995b, Sobel & Davanipour 1996).

Preliminary clinical trials with devices that shield against electromagnetic pollution show relief from a wide range of symptoms, suggesting that those problems may actually be caused or aggravated by electromagnetic pollution (Abraham, personal communication 1998). Whether these correlations will stand up to long-term research is unknown, but enough information is available on electromagnetic bioeffects to have led the US government to warn that prudent avoidance is a good policy until more is learned. At present we do not know what constitutes a 'safe limit' for electromagnetic field exposure. It is interesting that the Russian standard for maximum safe microwave exposure to avoid changes in brain activity is 1000 times less than the US legal maximum.

Low cost detectors of magnetic fields are available, and these devices are invaluable for those who wish to get a better appreciation of the fields present in their homes and workplaces. (A list of suppliers is given in Appendix I.) One of these devices (TriField from AlphaLab) is reasonably inexpensive and combines magnetic, electric, and radio/microwave detectors. The magnetic section has three detecting coils oriented in the three directions of space, which is important. With such devices, one can locate the 'hot spots' in the home and work environment, such as near electric blankets and heaters, fluorescent lights, light dimmers, microwave ovens with bad seals, cellular phones, computers, televisions, transformers, and motors in devices such as refrigerators and clocks. Sometimes moving furniture, cribs, or beds a short distance can significantly reduce long-term exposure.

Some people have taken steps to rewire their homes and workplaces to reduce the levels of 50 or 60 Hz magnetic fields. Simple changes in wiring configuration can make an enormous difference in the levels of magnetic fields in the home (Maxey 1991). However, Abraham (personal communication 1998) has cautioned that any method of field cancellation, such as twisting conductors together, can lead to the generation of undetectable 50 or 60 Hz scalar waves that could also have serious health effects. Obviously we have much to learn about our electromagnetic environment and its relations to therapeutics.

Avoidance of geopathic stress is also important. Hall (1997) presents some techniques, and dowsers are also a good source of suggestions.

Therapists are being introduced to a variety of devices that are promoted as shields against electromagnetic pollution. The consumer must be cautioned, however, that it is easy to be deceived in a situation where the effects are invisible and unmeasurable, and benefits are subjective. At present, the best way to assess such devices is by testing on a person who has electromagnetic sensitivity. This may seem unscientific, but there is a good precedent for it. Many of the important discoveries in biology began with sensitive biological assays, in which the strength of an unknown compound or other factor is estimated by testing it on a living system. This is called a bioassay (e.g. Glass 1973). The 'confrontation-neutralization technique' used by Choy and colleagues (1987) to study electrical sensitivities in allergy patients is a form of bioassay. The construction of an effective shield against electromagnetic effects is technically challenging, and will be greatly facilitated when reliable detectors of scalar waves have been developed.

Some conclusions

To the biologist, the advent of the electronic age represents a major evolutionary event, a dramatic step into the unknown. Developments in electricity and electronics have greatly expanded the limits of what humans can achieve. But advances often have unanticipated costs. Some of the scientists who did the early research on radioactivity, X-rays, and microwaves lost their lives because of the cumulative effects of exposure to the energies they had discovered.

We have introduced a wide spectrum of invisible and potentially dangerous factors into our environment. Physicists continue to calculate how these energies may or may not influence living systems, but the biological concepts upon which they base their calculations are often rudimentary and inaccurate. Living tissue is far more sophisticated than any material physicists work with in the laboratory. Living tissue has remarkable properties that continue to astonish us. The truth is that we simply will not know the long-term biological effects of electromagnetic technologies for several generations. We are participants in a long-term study, with an unknown outcome.

There is reliable evidence that electromagnetic fields are a double-edged sword. Some frequencies are not good for you, others can stimulate healing. Some of the negative effects are uncomfortable, others are life-threatening. The research on cells in culture is particularly valuable in documenting the biological effects of electromagnetic fields at the cellular level. At the same time, this research has important implications for energetic bodyworkers by revealing the sensitive regulatory pathways in living tissues. It now appears that a minute field oscillating at 50 or 60 Hz can be harmful, while a field of similar strength but lower in frequency (e.g. 2, 7, 10, and 15 Hz) can stimulate healing of tissues such as nerve, bone, ligament, and capillaries, respectively (see Chs 6 and 7).

References

Abraham G 1998 Potential shields against electromagnetic pollution: Synchroton Scalar Synchronizer. Optimox Corporation, PO Box 3378, Torrance, CA 90510-3378. Tel: 800-223-1601

Afilani T L 1998 Device and method using dielectrokinesis to locate entities. US Patent 5,748,088

Aharonov Y, Bohm E 1959 Significance of electromagnetic potentials in the quantum theory. Physical Reviews 115(3):485–491

Alexander G J, Gray R 1972 Induction of convulsive seizures in sound sensitive albino mice: response to various signal frequencies: 1. Proceedings of the Society for Experimental Biology and Medicine 140(4):1284–1288

Bellossi A, DeCertaines J, Bernard A M 1985 Is there an association between myocardial infarction and geomagnetic activity? International Journal of Biometeorology 29(1):1–6

Bennett W R 1994 Health and low-frequency electromagnetic fields. Yale University Press, New Haven

Benveniste J 1998 From 'water memory effects' to 'digital biology.' On the web at: http://www.digibio.com/

Best S T 1984 Laying it on the power line. Guardian, Oct 24, 1984

Best S T 1988 The electropollution effect. Journal of Alternative and Complementary Medicine (May):17, 18, 26, 30, 34, 43

Brewitt B 1996 Quantitative analysis of electrical skin conductance in diagnosis and current views of bioelectric medicine. Journal of Naturopathic Medicine 6(1):66-75

Brewitt B 1999 Electromagnetic medicine and HIV/AIDS treatment: clinical data and hypothesis for mechanism of action. In: Standish L J, Calabrese C, Galatino M L (eds) AIDS and alternative medicine: the current state of the science. Harcourt Brace, New York

Brown F A Jr 1973 Biological rhythms. In: Prosser C L (ed) Comparative Animal Physiology, 3rd edn. W B Saunders, Philadelphia, ch 10, pp 429–456

Bureau Y R, Persinger M A, Parker G H 1996 Effect of enhanced geomagnetic activity on hypothermia and mortality in rats. International Journal of Biometeorology 39(4):197–200

Burr H S 1957 Harold Saxton Burr. Yale Journal of Biology and Medicine 30(3):161–167

Chibrikin V M, Samovichev E G, Kashinskaya I V et al 1995 Dynamics of social processes and geomagnetic activity, 1: periodic components of variations in the number of recorded crimes in Moscow. Biofizika 40(5):1050–1053

Choy R V S, Monro J A, Smith C W 1987 Electrical sensitivities in allergy patients. Clinical Ecology 4(3):93–102

Conesa J 1995 Relationship between isolated sleep paralysis and geomagnetic influences: a case study. Perceptual and Motor Skills 80(3/2):1263–1273

De Matteis G, Vellante M, Marrelli A, Villante U, Santalucia P, Tuzi P, Perncipe M 1994 Geomagnetic activity, humidity, temperature and headache: is there any correlation? Headache 34(1):41–43

Di Perri R 1972 Photoprecipitable epilepsy: clinical observations and pathogenetic considerations. Acta Neurolgia (Napoli) 27(5):429–442

Dossey L 1993 Healing words: the power of prayer and the practice of medicine. Harper Collins, San Francisco

Dubrov A P 1978 The geomagnetic field and life: geomagnetobiology. Plenum Press, New York

Fellows L 1997 Opening up the 'black box.' International Journal of Alternative and Complementary Medicine 15(8):9–13

Foster H 1975 Letter. Photic fit near a helicopter. Lancet 2(7926):186

Gauquelin M 1966 Effets biologiques des champs magnétiques. Anné Biologique 11–12:595–611

Gauquelin M 1974 The cosmic clocks. Avon Books, New York

Gelinas R C 1984 Apparatus and method for transfer of information by means of a curl-free magnetic vector potential field. US Patent No 4,432,098

Glass G E (ed) 1973 Bioassay techniques and environmental chemistry. Ann Arbor Science, Ann Arbor, MI

Grigor'ev IuG 1995 Mild geomagnetic field as a risk factor in work in screened buildings. Meditsina Truda Promyshlennaya Ekologiya 0(4):7–12

Grinberg-Zylberbaum J, Delaflor M, Sanchez Arellano M E, Guevara M A, Perez M 1992 Human communication and the electrophysiological activity of the brain. Subtle Energies 3(3):25–43

Grinberg-Zylberbaum J, Delaflor M, Attie L, Goswami A 1994 The Einstein–Podolsky–Rosen paradox in the brain: the transferred potential. Physics Essays 7(4):422–428

Hainsworth L B 1983 The effect of geophysical phenomena on human health. Speculations in Science and Technology 6(5):439–444

Hall A 1997 Water, electricity and health: protecting yourself from electrostress at home and work. Hawthorn Press, Stroud, Gloucestershire

Harland J D, Liburdy R P 1997 Environmental magnetic fields inhibit the antiproliferative action of tamoxifen and melatonin in a human breast cancer cell line. Bioelectromagnetics. 18(8):555–562

Imry Y, Webb R A 1989 Quantum interference and the Aharonov–Bohm effect: these counterintuitive effects play important roles in the theory of electromagnetic interactions, in solid-state physics and possibly in the development of new microelectronic devices. Scientific American 260(4):56–62

Jackson J D 1975 Classical electrodynamics, 2nd edn. John Wiley, New York

Jacobs R 1997 21st century medicine. Kindred Spirit 3(10):37–40

Jones W H S 1948 Hippocrates. Harvard University Press, Cambridge, Massachusetts, vol 1, pp 73, 115

Kay R W 1994 Geomagnetic storms: association with incidence of depression as measured by hospital admission. British Journal of Psychiatry 164(3):403–409

Knox E G, Armstrong E, Lancashire R, Wall M, Haynes R 1979 Heart attacks and geomagnetic activity. Nature 281(5732):564–565

Kotleba J, Bielek J, Glos J et al 1973 Possible effect of the geomagnetic field on human sleep. Ceskoslovenska Fysiologie. 22(5):459–460

Lednev V V 1991 Possible mechanism for the influence of weak magnetic fields on biological systems. Bioelectromagnetics 12:71–75

Liburdy R P 1992 Calcium signaling in lymphocytes and ELF fields: evidence for an electric field metric and a site of interaction involving the calcium ion channel. FEBS Letters 301(1):53–59

Liburdy R P 1996 Electromagnetic fields and cellular systems: signal transduction, cell growth and proliferation. In: Ueno S (ed) Biological effects of magnetic and electromagnetic fields. Plenum Press, New York, ch 6, p 85

Liburdy R P, Vanek P F Jr 1985 Microwaves and the cell membrane, II: temperature, plasma, and oxygen mediate microwave-induced membrane permeability in the erythrocyte. Radiation Research 102(2):190–205

Liburdy R P, Wyant A 1984 Radiofrequency radiation and the immune system, part 3: in vitro effects on human immunoglobin and on murine T- and B-lymphocytes. International Journal of Radiation Biology and Related Studies in Physics, Chemistry and Medicine 46(1):67–81

Liburdy R P, Rowe A W, Vanek P F Jr 1988 Microwaves and the cell membrane, IV: protein shedding in the human erythrocyte: quantitative analysis by high-performance liquid chromatography. Radiation Research 114(3):500–514

Liburdy R P, Sloma T R, Sokolic R, Yaswen P 1993a ELF magnetic fields, breast cancer, and melatonin: 60 Hz fields block melatonin's oncostatic action on ER+ breast cancer cell proliferation. Journal of Pineal Research 14(2):89–97

Liburdy R P, Callahan D E, Harland J, Dunham E, Sloma T R, Yaswen P 1993b Experimental evidence for 60 Hz magnetic fields operating through the signal transduction cascade: effects on calcium influx and c-MYC mRNA induction. FEBS Letters 334(3):301–308

Lin J C (ed) 1994 Advances in electromagnetic fields in living systems, vol 1. Plenum Press, New York

Lin J C (ed) 1997 Advances in electromagnetic fields in living systems, vol 2. Plenum Press, New York

Lipa B J, Sturrock P A, Rogot E 1976 Search for correlation between geomagnetic disturbances and mortality. Nature 259(5541):302–304

Maxey E S 1991 A lethal subtle energy. Subtle Energies 2(2):55–70

Michon A L, Persinger M A 1997 Experimental simulation of the effects of increased geomagnetic activity upon nocturnal seizures in epileptic rats. Neurosciences Letters 224(1):53–56

Michon A, Koren S A, Persinger M A 1996 Attempts to simulate the association between geomagnetic activity and spontaneous seizures in rats using experimentally generated magnetic fields. Perceptual and Motor Skills 82(2):619–626

Mikulecky M, Moravclova G, Czanner S 1996 Lunisolar tidal waves, geomagnetic activity and epilepsy in the light of multivariate coherence. Brazilian Journal of Medical and Biological Research 29(8):1069–1072

Moore-Ede M C, Campbell S S, Reiter R J 1992 Electromagnetic fields and circadian rhythmicity. Birkhäuser, Boston

Olariu S, Popescu II 1985 The quantum effects of electromagnetic fluxes. Reviews of Modern Physics 57:339–436

Oschman J L (2000) Energy medicine: the new paradigm. In: Charman R (ed) Complementary therapies for physical therapists: a theoretical and clinical exploration. Butterworth Heinemann, Oxford, introductory chapter

Peat F D 1987 Synchronicity: the bridge between matter and mind. Bantam Books, Toronto

Persinger M A 1996 Enhancement of limbic seizures by nocturnal application of experimental magnetic fields that simulate the magnitude and morphology of increases in geomagnetic activity. International Journal of Neuroscience 86(3–4):271–280

Persinger M A, Krippner S 1993 Dream ESP experiments and geomagnetic activity. In: Kane B, Millay J, Brown D (eds) Silver threads: 25 years of parapsychology research. Praeger, Westport, Connecticut, ch 3, pp 39–53

Persinger M A, Psych C 1995 Sudden unexpected death in epileptics following sudden, intense, increases in geomagnetic activity: prevalence of effect and potential mechanisms. International Journal of Biometeorology 38(4):180–187

Persinger M A, Richards M 1995 Vestibular experiences of humans during brief periods of partial sensory deprivation are enhanced when daily geomagnetic activity exceeds 15–20 nT. Neurosciences Letters 194(1–2):69–72

Polikarpov N A 1996 The relationship of the indices of solar-geomagnetic activity and the autofluctuations in the biological properties of Staphylococcus aureus 209 subcultures in vitro. Zhurnal Mikrobiologil Epidemiologii Immunobiologii (1):27–30

Presman A S 1970 Electromagnetic fields and life. Plenum Press, New York

Rajaram M, Mitra S 1981 Correlation between convulsive seizure and geomagnetic activity. Neuroscience Letters 24:187–191

Rein G 1998 Biological effects of quantum fields and their role in the natural healing process. Frontier Perspectives 7(1):16–23

Reiter R 1953 Neuere Untersuchungen zum Problem der Wetterabhängigkeit des Menschen. Archiv für Meterologie, Geophysik und Bioclimatologie B4:327 [For a review of Reiter's work in English, see König H L 1974 Behavioral changes in human subjects associated with ELF electric fields. In: Persinger M A (ed) ELF and VLF electromagnetic field effects. Plenum Press, New York, pp 81–99. Also, see Moore-Ede M C,

Campbell S S, Reiter R J 1992 Electromagnetic fields and circadian rhythmicity. Birkhäuser, Boston]

Rohrlich F 1983 Facing quantum mechanical reality. Science 221(4617):1251–1255

Rolf I P 1962 Structural integration: gravity: an unexplored factor in a more human use of human beings. Journal of the Institute for the Comparative Study of History, Philosophy and the Sciences 1:3–20 [Available from the Rolf Institute, Boulder, Colorado 800-530-8875]

St Pierre L, Persinger M A 1998 Geophysical variables and behavior, LXXXIV: quantitative increases in group aggression in male epileptic rats during increases in geomagnetic activity. Perceptual and Motor Skills 86(3/2):1392–1394

Schienle A, Stark R, Vaitl D 1998 Biological effects of very low frequency (VLF) atmospherics in humans: a review. Journal of Scientific Exploration 12(3):455–468

Seymour P 1988 Astrology: the evidence of science. Penguin, London

Smith C W 1987 Electromagnetic effects in humans. In: Fröhlich H (ed) Biological coherence and response to external stimuli. Springer-Verlag, Berlin, pp 205–232

Smith C W, Best S 1989 Electromagnetic man: health and hazard in the electrical environment. J M Dent, London

Sobel E, Davanipour Z 1996 Electromagnetic field exposure may cause increased production of amyloid beta and eventually lead to Alzheimer's disease. Neurology 47(6):1477–1481

Sobel E, Davanipour Z, Sulkava R, et al 1995a Occupational exposure to electromagnetic fields: a possible risk factor for Alzheimer's disease. In: Iqbal K, Mortimer J A, Winblad B, Wisniewski H M (eds) Research advances in Alzheimer's disease and related disorders. John Wiley, Chichester

Sobel E, Dunn M, Davanipour Z, Qian Z, Chui H C 1995b Elevated risk of Alzheimer's disease among workers with likely electromagnetic field exposure. American Journal of Epidemiology 142(5):515–524

Stocks P 1925 High barometer and sudden deaths. British Medical Journal 2:1188

Stoupel E 1993 Sudden cardiac deaths and ventricular extrasystoles on days with four levels of geomagnetic activity. Journal of Basic Clinical Physiology and Pharmacology 4(4):357–366

Stoupel E, Martfel J, Rotenberg Z 1991 Admissions of patients with epileptic seizures (E) and dizziness (D) related to geomagnetic and solar activity levels: differences in female and male patients. Medical Hypotheses 36(4):384–388

Stoupel E, Goldenfeld M, Shimshoni M, Siegel R 1993 Intraocular pressure (IOP) in relation to four levels of daily geomagnetic and extreme yearly solar activity. International Journal of Biometeorology 37(1):42–45

Stoupel E, Martfel J, Rotenberg Z 1994 Paroxysmal atrial fibrillation and stroke (cerebrovascular accidents) in males and females above and below age 65 on days of different geomagnetic activity levels. Journal of Basic Clinical Physiology and Pharmacology 5(3–4):315–329

Stoupel E, Wittenberg C, Zabludowski J, Boner G 1995 Ambulatory blood pressure monitoring in patients with hypertension on days of high and low geomagnetic activity. Journal of Human Hypertension 9(4):293–294

Szent-Györgyi A 1957 Bioenergetics. Academic Press, New York

Tambiev A E, Medvedev S D, Egorova E V 1995 The effect of geomagnetic disturbances on the functions of attention and memory. Aviakosmicheskaia Ekologicheskaia Meditsina 29(3):43–45

Teneforde T S, Kaune W T 1987 Interaction of extremely low frequency electric and magnetic fields with humans. Health Physics 53(6):585–606

Tesla N 1904 Transmission of energy without wires. Scientific American Supplement 57:237

Usenko G A, Panin L E 1993 Blood system reactions in flight operators with high and low levels of anxiousness during geomagnetic disturbances. Aviakosmicheskaia Ekologicheskaia Meditsina 27(2):39–44

Valet J-P, Meynadier L 1993 Geomagnetic field intensity and reversals during the past four million years. Nature 366(6452):234–238

Venkataraman K 1976 Epilepsy and solar activity: an hypothesis. Neurology India 24:148–152

Ward R R 1971 The living clocks. Alfred A Knopf, New York, p 64 et seq

Watanabe Y, Hillman D C, Otsuka K, Bingham C, Breus T K, Cornelissen G, Halberg F 1994 Cross-spectral coherence between geomagnetic disturbance and human cardiovascular variables at non-societal frequencies. Chronobiologia 21(3–4):265–272

Wever R 1968 Einfluss Schwacher Elektro-magnetischer Felder auf die Circadiane Periodik des Menschen. Naturwissenschaften 55:29–32 [For a summary of Wever's work in English, see Wever R 1974 ELF-effects on human circadian rhythms. In: Persinger M A (ed) ELF and VLF electromagnetic field effects. Plenum Press, New York, pp 101–144]

Whittaker E T 1903 On the partial differential equations of mathematical physics. Mathematische Annalen 57:333–355

Whittaker E T 1904 On an expression of the electromagnetic field due to electrons by means of two scalar potential functions. Proceedings of the London Mathematical Society 1:367–372

Woodhouse M B 1996 Paradigm wars: worldviews for a new age. Frog, Berkeley, CA

Yost M G, Liburdy R P 1992 Time-varying and static magnetic fields act in combination to alter calcium signal transduction in the lymphocyte. FEBS Letters 296(2):117–122

Ynduráin FJ 1983 Quantum chromodynamics: an introduction to the theory of quarks and gluons. Springer–Verlag, New York

15 ▸ Conclusions: is energy medicine the medicine of the future?

Prematurity

A discovery is premature if its implications cannot be connected by a series of simple logical steps to canonical, or generally accepted, knowledge.
G. Stent (1972)

Some discoveries are made before their time, and simply cannot be integrated into contemporary thought. Concepts of 'life energy' and 'healing energy' have surfaced many times over the centuries. Until recently, these concepts have been classic examples of prematurity.

This situation has now changed. A firm basis has been established for energetic phenomena previously regarded as impossible or unlikely. Scientists have developed more than adequate measurable and logical connections between biological energy fields and generally accepted scientific knowledge. The key discoveries have been made in the course of ordinary science, in a wide range of disciplines, following traditional methods and logic. Because of the traditional bias against any examination of topics like 'healing energy' and 'life force', a veritable scientific revolution has taken place without attracting any interest in the academic community. Hopefully this book will introduce the subject to those in the biomedical research community who are open-minded enough to consider new possibilities for research and clinical applications.

The following is a synthesis of the key advances discussed in this book:

◆ Early in the 20th century it was discovered that the various organs in the body produce electrical fields that can be detected on the skin. This led to important clinical tools such as electrocardiography and electroencephalography.

◆ When electric currents flow through tissues, the laws of physics dictate that magnetic fields must be created in the surrounding region, but it was not until the 1950s that instruments were developed to detect them. The SQUID magnetometer is now being used in medical research laboratories around the world to map the ever-changing biomagnetic fields produced by various organs. This has led to new clinical tools such as magnetocardiography and magnetoencephalography.

◆ Medical researchers have explored the application of electric and magnetic fields to stimulate healing. Pulsing magnetic fields are particularly effective. Remarkably, pulsing magnetic fields can also be emitted from the human hand under certain conditions. These natural emissions sweep up and down through the range of frequencies with demonstrated therapeutic effectiveness. The emitted frequencies are influenced by geophysical rhythms, which can entrain brain waves and other biological rhythms. This correlates with the discovery that living systems respond to external energy fields at or near the limits imposed by the laws of physics (Bialek 1987). Once information has been extracted from the environment, the living matrix and the nervous system can process the information with virtually no addition of noise.

◆ Sensitive photometers and thermographic imaging techniques have enabled scientists to map the patterns of light and heat emitted by cells, tissues, organs and the whole body.

◆ Spectroscopic methods reveal the energy emissions and adsorptions of molecules, and thereby reveal the roles of energy fields in molecular processes, including hormone–receptor, antibody–antigen and allergic interactions. Spectroscopy provides the basis for pharmacology, homeopathy, aromatherapy, and herbal medicines.

◆ Cell biologists are recognizing that regulations involve more than nerve impulses and hormones. The nuclear, cytoplasmic, and extracellular matrices form a continuous and interconnected communication system. The solid state, electronic, photonic, and vibratory properties of this living matrix continuum play key roles in integration of functions, including injury repair and defense against disease. Tensegrity concepts explain how the various forms of energy are absorbed and conducted throughout the framework of the body, affecting all cells. Movements, tensions, and other energies conducted through this system interact with metabolism and the genetic material. Vibrations of living matrix molecules are affected by cellular activities, growth factors, carcinogenesis, and emotional states.

◆ Some of the vibratory phenomena in the living matrix are coherent or laser-like in nature. The high degree of regularity or crystallinity found in many tissues goes hand in hand with the regularity or coherence of the energy systems.

On the basis of what is now known about the roles of electrical, magnetic, elastic, acoustic, thermal, gravitational, and photonic energies in living systems, it appears that there is no single 'life force' or 'healing energy' in living systems. Instead, there are many energetic systems in the living body, and many ways of influencing those systems. What we refer to as the 'living state' and as 'health' are all of these systems, both known and unknown, functioning collectively, cooperatively, synergistically. The debate about whether there is such a thing as a healing energy or life force is being replaced with study of the interactions between biological energy fields, structures, and functions.

Complementing these scientific discoveries is a long history of empirical evidence and clinical technique developed by therapists of various kinds, who have honed their perception and intuition to gain deep insights into living systems. The growing popularity of bodywork, energetic and movement therapies is leading us to a synthesis of ideas that will be beneficial to all.

At the same time, the discovery that living systems respond to minute electromagnetic fields has led to concern that electromagnetic pollution in our environment may be hazardous to health. Some physicists have taken the position that there is little or no such danger, based upon their deep understanding of electromagnetic phenomena. The problem with this is that while electromagnetism has been widely studied by physicists, study of biological electromagnetism has just begun. The problem was articulated years ago by physicist Werner Heisenberg: 'Something has to be added to the laws of physics and chemistry before the biological phenomena can be completely understood.'

Emissions from the hands of therapists

Of all of the discoveries summarized above, the most tenuous, and yet the most exciting, is the discovery of the huge biomagnetic fields emitted from the hands of therapists of various kinds. If the phenomenon is as robust and repeatable as it seems, its documentation, by Zimmerman (1985) and Seto et al (1992) (see Chs 6 and 7), will take an important place in the history of medical biology.

The finding is tenuous in that it has not been widely replicated. Moreover, it would be useful to have a detailed spectral analysis of the emissions from the hands. From the information presented so far, we would expect to find signals representing a wide range of molecular, cellular, tissue, organ, and whole body activities. The magnetic emissions are probably accompanied by a mix of acoustic, photonic, thermal, and other forms of energy.

As discussed in Chapter 6, the phenomenon was originally described in the context of therapeutic touch and was confirmed for QiGong and other martial arts and contemplative practices. Figure 15.1 compares the strengths of natural and artificial magnetic fields from a variety of sources.

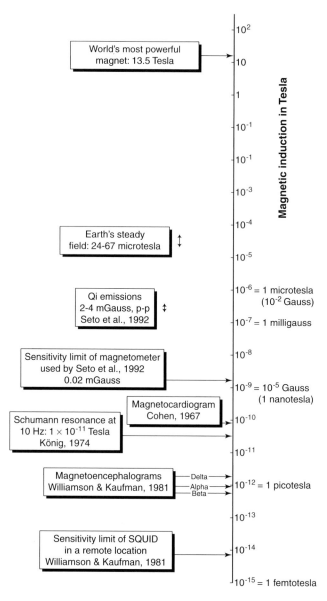

Fig. 15.1   Comparison of the strengths of natural and artificial magnetic fields from a variety of sources. The field strength of the world's most powerful magnet data from a report in *Science News* (Wu 1997).

Practitioners of bodywork, energetic and movement therapies have daily and remarkable encounters with the therapeutic effects of energy fields. There is a growing body of evidence for the effectiveness of these methods. However, the impact of even the most carefully controlled studies can be compromised if the findings cannot be connected logically to generally accepted biomedical paradigms. For the biologist, there is a profoundly interesting question: 'Can humans proactively, or self-consciously, or intentionally change the margins of their biology in medically significant ways by what they think and feel?' (Foss 1997). Another fundamental biological problem is the 'crisis in energetics' that continues to plague the academic field of bioenergetics (Green 1973).

An energetic perspective is enabling us to restate important but confusing questions that have been kept at the fringes of science for a long time. The remainder of the book takes up some of the topics that are worthy of further research.

Amplification

In Chapter 2 it was mentioned that magnetic brain waves associated with the sensory and motor cortex become stronger when an action is practiced again and again, as occurs when one rehearses with a musical instrument. Similar changes may occur with repeated practice of various 'hands-on' therapies. It would not be surprising if the various yogic, martial arts, and contemplative practices also lead to stronger and more coherent biomagnetic fields.

While more research is needed, the most logical explanation for amplification is that the waves of electrical and magnetic activity from the brain are amplified as they pass through the peripheral tissues. Vibrating molecules throughout the body may become cooperatively entrained with the brain rhythms. As more and more molecules within the crystalline living matrix become vibrationally entrained, the fields get stronger.

Bodywork and other repetitive practices such as yoga, QiGong, tai chi, meditation, therapeutic touch, etc. may gradually lead to more structural coherence (crystallinity) in the tissues, facilitating both the detection and radiation of energy fields (Oschman & Oschman 1997). Arrays of water molecules associated with the macromolecules are probably involved as well.

The process has been described as the formation of 'coherence domains' in liquid crystal arrays (Sermonti 1995). The mechanism involves the stabilization of the positional and orientational order of millions of rod-shaped molecules, as in cell membranes, connective tissues, DNA, muscle, the cytoskeleton, the myelin sheath of nerves, and sensory cells (Oschman 1997). Stabilization spreads from molecule to molecule, throughout the system. Del Guidice (1993) describes the process as one in which individual molecules 'lose their individual identity, cannot be separated, move together as if performing a choral ballet, and are kept in phase by an electromagnetic field which arises from the same ballet'.

Years ago, Harold Saxton Burr made a related statement: 'the pattern or organization of any biological system is established by an electrical field which is at the same time determined by its components and determines the orientation of the components. The field maintains the pattern in the midst of a flux of components. This is the mechanism whose outcome is wholeness, organization, continuity' (Burr 1972) (see Ch. 1).

A related explanation for amplification arises from the word 'laser'(an acronym for light amplification by stimulated emission of radiation). Lasers *amplify* light by recycling some of the coherent or highly organized energy back into the system, where it can stimulate even more coherent emissions. The energy fed back into the system maintains the high rate and order of the atomic vibrations that give rise to the radiation. Crystalline components of the living matrix, such as the collagen arrays in tendons, ligaments, and bones, and the arrays of lipids in cell membranes, probably act as coherent resonant molecular broadcasting systems.

Electronics engineers know that a transmitting antenna works best when its length corresponds with the wavelength of the signal being broadcasted. And the same length is also ideal for the receiving antenna. Hence it is possible that various deep tissue, stretching, nutritional, contemplative, and other practices of therapists and their clients gradually modify their tissues in ways that stabilize the 'coherence domains' within their tissues, enhancing their ability both to detect and to radiate coherent energy. Other biophysical mechanisms may be involved:

◆ Superconduction and superfluidity: Pauling (1936) and London (1950) suggested that the electron currents around benzene rings are superconductive currents. Little (1964) demonstrated that biomolecules should, in principle, superconduct at body temperatures. Demonstrations of organic superconduction have been reported by Cope (1975, 1978) and by Wolf and colleagues (Wolf 1976, Wolf & Halpern 1976, Wolf et al 1976).

◆ Phonon super-radiance: Bialek (1984) has described how a polymer system, such as the macromolecular arrays in living tissues, can be driven into a large scale coherent oscillation. A number of physicists raised objections to this hypothesis, but Del Giudice and Preparata (1990) showed how super-radiance arises as a consequence of the quantum properties of 'condensed matter'.

◆ Superfluorescence: Bonifacio et al (1984) have described how arrays of Josephson junctions, which have been predicted to exist in living systems, can produce a coupled resonant radiation field.

◆ Plasmas: Sedlak (1971, 1979, 1982) and Roffey (1993, 1994) suggested that the magnetic sensitivity of living systems is, in part, due to a plasma state that exists in living matter.

In summary, quantum consideration of highly regular arrays of molecules, as occur throughout the living body, gives rise to a number of possible explanations for remarkable energetic phenomena. Some have suggested that there are undiscovered natural forces or 'subtle energies' (defined as 'delicate' or 'refined'). While this is possible, we have enough information to develop at least a partial picture of how living systems use known forces, and how therapists of various kinds use these energies to stimulate healing. We explore this below in more detail, with some specific examples, beginning with the nervous system.

The dual nervous system

The nervous system is a fundamental energy system in the body. Its operation is studied by measuring electrical fields generated during the transmission of nerve impulses. As electric currents always give rise to magnetic fields, the nervous system is also a source of some of the biomagnetic fields present within and around the organism. Moreover, the nervous system regulates all muscular movements, and is therefore key to converting thoughts into energetic actions (defined in physics as the kinetic energy of movements, gravitational potential energy of objects lifted, elastic energy of impacts and vibrations such as sound and heat).

Neurophysiologists focus most of their attention on the 'classical' nervous system, composed of the neurons that conduct information from place to place as electrical impulses. The 'neuron doctrine' holds that all functions of the nervous system result from the activities of the neurons. Hence integration of brain function, memory, and even consciousness have been assumed to arise from the massive interconnectivity of the neurons.

This is a partial view because it neglects another energetic and informational system consisting of the perineural connective tissue system, which constitutes more than half of the cells in the brain (the prefix 'peri-' means about, around, encircling, or enclosing). Perineural cells surround each neuron in the brain, and follow every peripheral nerve to its termination (inset, Fig. 15.2).

Robert O. Becker has been a pioneer in exploring the functions of the perineural system and its relationship with the semiconducting matrix that forms and surrounds it. To document the properties of this system, Becker refers to a 'dual nervous system,' consisting of the classical digital (all-or-none) nerve network, and the perineural analogue network, which regulates wound healing and tissue repair. Figure 15.2 illustrates the dual nervous system and summarizes the properties of its two components.

From the perspective of regulatory biology, the neural and perineural systems are virtually opposite in character. An individual neuron is capable of conducting a stimulus from one precise point to another, such as when a motor nerve triggers a particular muscle to contract, or when a sensory neuron conveys information from a particular receptor to the sensory cortex. While nerves are not electrically or magnetically insulated, and there is some 'information leakage' into surrounding tissues (Oschman 1990), the neural impulse is propagated some distance without decrement (loss of energy) from its site of origin to a very precise point (e.g. a synapse) within the neural network.

A direct current control system

In contrast to the neuronal system, the perineural connective tissue generates slower moving waves of direct current that flow throughout the organism, affecting every part. The primary pacemaker is the brain wave oscillation that spreads throughout the brain, and then through the perineural system, to every part of the body that is innervated. Moreover, as the brain is richly vascularized, and blood is an excellent conductor of electricity, the brain waves also flow through the circulatory system. Hence brain waves, electricity from the heart and other muscles, and signals from other organs get mixed together in the circulatory system.

Brain waves are modified or modulated by smaller fields associated with particular activities, such as those involved in sensation, movement, and thought. Like a pebble thrown into a pond, any electrical or magnetic activity or perturbation is propagated throughout the system along with the larger waves.

If one were devising a cybernetic network to regulate the operation of a system as intricate as the human body, it would make sense to employ both kinds of communication represented by the dual nervous system. Point-to-point transmission allows for very precise control of specific activities and precise sensory feedbacks. In contrast, the perineural system does not have a specific target – it delivers regulatory messages to every part. It is a global system, integrating and regulating processes throughout the organism.

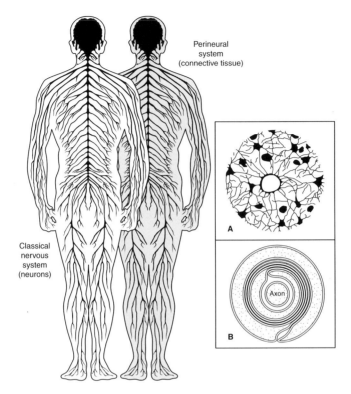

Fig. 15.2 The dual nervous system. If a way were devised to dissolve all of the nerves in the brain and throughout the body, it would appear to the naked eye that nothing was missing. The brain and the spinal cord and all of the peripheral nerves would be intact down to their smallest terminations. This is because the central nervous system is composed of two separate types of cells: the nerve cells, or 'neurons', and the 'perineural cells'. (Becker 1990a, 1990b, 1991) The 'classical' nervous system is composed of neurons conducting information from place to place as electrical impulses. The signals are digital or 'all or none' in nature. Signals may be individual spikes, or trains of pulses. Digital systems provide high speed, high volume information transfer. In terms of evolution and phylogeny, this nervous system is a relatively recent innovation. This system is responsible for sensation and movement, and communications are 'point-to-point'. In contrast, the perineural nervous system is composed of perineural cells that conduct information from place to place as relatively slowly varying direct currents. These slow waves are analog rather than digital. Analog systems cannot transmit large amounts of data, but are ideally suited for precise control of individual functions. Some of these oscillations are maintained by pacemakers (e.g. brain waves). In terms of evolution and phylogeny, the perineural system is ancient. This system is responsible for overall regulation of the classical nervous system, and for regulating wound healing and injury repair. Instead of point-to-point signaling, information propagated by this system spreads throughout the body. The insets show examples of perineural cells. **A** Fibrous astrocytes with end feet around a small blood vessel **B** A Schwann cell surrounding an axon in the peripheral nervous system. (Inset **A** from Glees 1955 Neurologia: Morphology and Function, with permission from Blackwell Science Ltd. Inset **B** is adapted from Fawcett 1994, Fig. 11.21, p. 335, with permission from Arnold.)

Most physiologists study point-to-point regulations, such as neural pathways or hormone–receptor interactions. Global or system-wide regulations are acknowledged to be important, but have received less attention, partly because of a lack of a theoretical basis for them. The historic mental block against the study of biological energetics has taken its toll on the study of regulations, because all messages are fundamentally reducible to energetic phenomena (Feynman 1996 discusses this in detail).

Becker's work on the perineural system and solid state communication in the living matrix has many clinical implications. He has presented evidence that the perineural system actually regulates the operation of the neurons, and not the reverse. The perineural system is involved in a number of important phenomena:

◆ The effects of geomagnetic fields on brain waves, which then affect animal activities such as navigation, psychiatric ward behavior, reaction time, and biological rhythms (Becker 1990a; Hamer 1965, 1969; Reiter 1953).

◆ The production of deep anesthesia by artificially reversing the fronto-occipital electric vector with a DC current (Becker 1991), and the production of the hypnotic state.

◆ Control of growth and regeneration.

◆ Control of injury repair. The perineural system is involved in the conduction of a slow wave, called the injury potential, away from a site of trauma. The injury potential plays a role in system-wide regulation, and coordination and integration of wound healing.

Energetic pulses precede actions: a basis for mental imaging and intention

Pulses of electric and magnetic energy begin in the brain *before* any movement occurs. This 'motor sequence' is the subject of much research around the world. Early work (Deecke et al 1969, 1976) identified four electrical components, and subsequent research (summarized by Okada 1983) describes the corresponding magnetic components that can be detected with the SQUID magnetometer.

The motor sequence modulates the electric and magnetic fields of the brain that spread throughout the body via the perineural DC analogue system.

Again, it makes sense that a living cybernetic network generates a set of signals that are spread out over time: first there are signals that prepare the system for action, then there are signals that trigger the action, and, finally, there are feedback signals that report that the action has been completed. The timing of this sequence for the flexion of the right index finger is shown in Figure 15.3. Awareness can arise in this unfoldment at a number of points, as we become conscious of the need for the act, of the act in process, and of its completion.

Related to this is an important phenomenon that is being investigated for its application in training for athletic events, dance, theatre, music, combat, and for healing work. Performers, therapists, and patients alike can benefit from *mental* rehearsals or internal imaging, without physically doing anything (e.g. Suinn 1985, Warner & McNeill 1988, Meyers et al 1996). The mechanisms involved have been unclear (Paivio 1985).

On the basis of the information presented in this book, there is a simple explanation. First, mental practice of movements sets up the anticipatory fields described above, without causing any muscles to move. Kasai et al (1997) refer to this as 'subthreshold muscle activity'. From Figure 15.3, we would expect imagery to produce the readiness potential and, possibly, the pre-motion potential, without the motor potential that triggers the movement. Mentally rehearsing an action sends information throughout the body, via the perineural and other conductive systems, to all of the relevant cells. This then leads to a 'preconditioning' of biochemical pathways, energy reserves, and patterns of information flow. Cells everywhere are then poised to work together at the instant of demand.

Many athletes, performers, and therapists of various kinds have described the profound experience of being totally prepared, present, and focused (see for example Murphy 1992). It is during these periods, sometimes referred to as 'the zone', that extraordinary accomplishments take place.

Many therapeutic schools emphasize the importance of intention: deciding in advance the goals they wish to attain for particular clients. This approach is based on the frequent experience that a vivid image of expectations facilitates change in that direction. Intention seems to be all the more effective when the client participates in it, as in directed movement therapies or image-based cancer treatments.

We have suggested that the effectiveness of various kinds of 'hands-on' bodywork can arise, in part, from the mutual entrainment of electrical and magnetic rhythms from therapist to client (Ch. 8). The 'anticipatory fields' described above may be an important component of this entrainment. Hence there is a physiological basis for the mental state of the practitioner 'preparing' the various parts of a client's body for work that is to be done later, or extending the work deeply into the tissues of the client to reach trauma that is deeply held, as in the 'trauma energetics' work of Redpath (see Ch. 8).

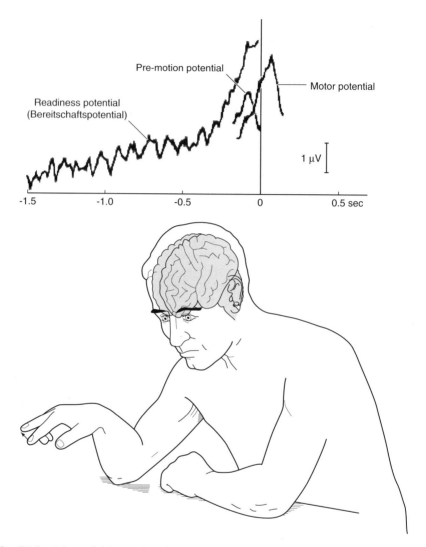

Fig. 15.3 Motor field associated with flexion of right index finger. The initiation and execution of a voluntary movement involves a sequence of activities in different parts of the brain. Four electrical components have been identified (Deecke et al 1969, 1976) and the corresponding magnetic components have been detected (reviewed by Okada 1983). At the top are shown the electrical recordings from different brain regions superimposed on the same time scale. The vertical line, 0 represents the onset of the actual movement as measured with an electromyogram. The slow 'readiness potential' or Bereitschaftspotential, begins as much as 1.5 seconds before the onset of the movement. This is followed by a pre-motion potential a few hundred milliseconds before the movement. The motor potential proper begins about 50 milliseconds before the movement. Not shown is the somatosensory or proprioceptive feedback potential, which follows the movement. (Taken from Okada 1983, Fig. 12.7.1, p. 423 and used with kind permission from Plenum Press.)

It is easy to be skeptical about the notion that the minute magnetic brain waves of a therapist could have any influence on cells and tissues throughout the body of a client. However, keep in mind that these magnetic fields are not as subtle as they might seem, because of the amplification effect (p. 221) and windowing (Fig. 13.1). Moreover, as we see below, there is a physical basis for the effects of biomagnetic fields on cells throughout the body, and the body of the person being touched.

The Hall effect and biomagnetic regulations

How can subtle variations in biomagnetic fields affect cells and tissues? A simple answer emerges from Becker's original research, indicating that the living matrix is a semiconductor network (Becker 1961). His experiments involved the Hall effect, named after a famous experiment performed in 1879 by physicist E. H. Hall. This effect distinguishes between ionic conduction and semiconduction. A magnetic field causes a current flowing in a semiconductor to veer off to one side, because a semiconductor contains a relatively small number of electrons, and they are very mobile (Fig. 15.4). Ionic conductance is different because there are many charge carriers and they are less mobile.

The degree of semiconduction is measured by the DC transverse Hall voltage, which is produced by a magnetic field positioned at right angles to the current flow. In studies on salamander limbs, Becker found Hall voltages indicative of semiconduction, rather than ionic currents. The Hall voltages increased during recovery from anesthesia, indicating that the semiconducting DC current correlates with the level of consciousness.

The Hall effect in semiconductors is one physical explanation of how magnetic effects are produced in the body. These effects can be either from iron magnets, or from the biomagnetic field of a therapist. The semiconducting Hall effect may also be involved in those situations where there is a conscious intention to entrain the rhythms of two or more individuals. The plasma concept described by Roffey (1993) may also be involved in the sensitivity of living systems to external magnetic fields.

The duality of the circulatory, skeletal, muscular, and other systems

While functions differ, the concept of the duality of the nervous system has implications for the other major systems in the body. For example, every blood vessel, from the arteries and veins down to the finest capillaries, is made of

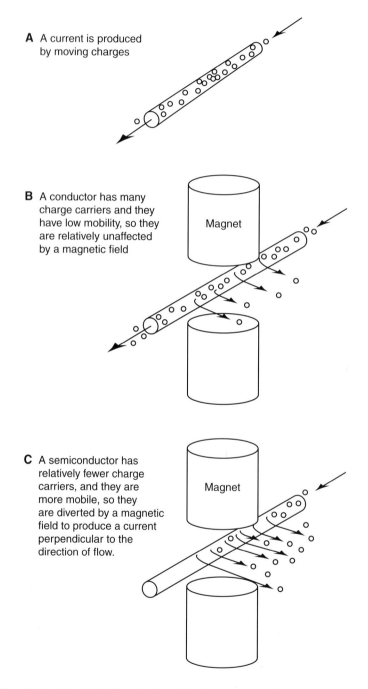

A A current is produced by moving charges

B A conductor has many charge carriers and they have low mobility, so they are relatively unaffected by a magnetic field

Magnet

C A semiconductor has relatively fewer charge carriers, and they are more mobile, so they are diverted by a magnetic field to produce a current perpendicular to the direction of flow.

Magnet

Fig. 15.4 The Hall effect distinguishes between conduction and semiconduction. (After Becker & Selden 1985, p. 113, reproduced with kind permission from Robert O. Becker MD.)

perivascular connective tissue. Like the perineural system, the perivascular system extends into every nook and cranny of the organism. Vascular tissue obviously functions as a conduit for the flow of blood. On the basis of the discoveries listed above we can also examine the perivascular system as a continuous communication system, with roles in regulation and physiological integration that go beyond plumbing. Electrical currents in the perivascular system are important in inflammation, haemostasis, and injury repair, and in carcinogenesis, in which vascular supplies to specific areas adjust to nourish a growing tumor.

Likewise, every bone in the body is surrounded by a periosteal connective tissue system. The bones have their obvious roles in support and movement, while the periosteal system has osteogenic potency (i.e. the ability to form new bone, such as occurs after a fracture). Moreover, bones have a very rich vascular supply, so the periosteal and perivascular systems are intimately connected.

The muscular system is also embedded in an intricate and interconnected perimysium, endomysium, and epimysium that merge together to form the tendons. While this connective tissue system is widely recognized for its role in conducting tensions generated by the muscles, therapists of various schools have come to recognize that it is also a communication medium, as well as the substance that gives overall form to the body (e.g. Varela & Frenk 1987). One function is in the regeneration and repair of damaged muscle (Mauro et al 1970) and the adaptation of muscles to functional demands (Guba et al 1981). Again, the musculature is extensively innervated and vascularized, so the other 'peri-' systems interdigitate with it.

Functions of the 'peri-' systems in regeneration and repair

In each of the examples given above, we make a distinction between the obvious primary function of a particular system – such as nerve, blood vessel, bone, or muscle – and the functions of the connective tissue system that surrounds and maintains it.

Each of the 'peri-' tissues surrounds or encloses one of the great systems of the body. We can refer to these tissues collectively as 'surrounding tissues'. Each of these surrounding tissues contains a sparse but active and important population of cells. These generative cells (fibroblasts, neuroblasts, myoblasts, osteoblasts, chondroblasts, etc.) form and continuously modify the extracellular matrix (ECM), and play key roles in injury repair.

Regeneration

Regeneration is the regrowth of missing or damaged tissues. Salamanders can completely regrow limbs, eyes, gut, spinal cord, half of the heart, and one-third of the brain tissue. This is accomplished by de-differentiation of all of the mature fibroblasts and other generative cells at the site of the injury. The generative cells are restored to their embryonic or totipotent state, so they can re-form any tissue in a process that resembles embryonic growth.

Becker's work on salamanders demonstrated that de-differentiation was accomplished by altering the electrical environment at the site of a wound. In essence, the repressed genes could be unlocked with extremely weak electrical fields (Becker & Selden 1985).

Until recently, regenerative healing in man has been limited to bone fractures. During research on critical infections in bone, Becker (1985, 1990b) discovered an electrochemical method that simultaneously controls bacterial infections and de-differentiates human fibroblasts to produce huge numbers of embryonic cells. Clinical trials revealed accelerated healing of skin, bone, and soft tissues, without scar formation. Becker reports that the method 'is useful in chronic, multiply infected wounds, acute wounds with major soft tissue and bone loss, and in ionizing radiation burns'. This extremely promising energetic therapy also de-differentiates and stops the growth of a variety of types of cancer cells.

These remarkable clinical results represent a breakthrough in both our theoretical and our practical understanding of the energetics of living systems. Below, we take a closer look at the energetic system involved.

Global interconnectedness of the fiber systems

The continuity or global interconnectedness of the living matrix is essential to the understanding of the body and the role of energetics in health and disease. The extracellular matrix (ECM) exerts specific and important influences upon cellular dynamics, just as much as hormones or neurotransmitters. Dramatic documentation of this fact comes from attempts to use hormones to induce normal differentiation of mammary tissue in vitro. These efforts were unsuccessful. However, when mammary cells are grown on the noncellular ECM of mammary glands, differentiation takes place and functional mammary tissue forms.

Hence the ECM actually regulates the genetic expression of the mammary cells (reviewed by Varela & Frenk 1987). Throughout the body, the ECM forms the intimate milieu of every cell and molecule. Its most important property, its interconnectedness, has not been appreciated.

The ECM has both local and global or systemic qualities. In an important conceptual paper, Varela & Frenk (1987) describe how these qualities interact. At every place in the body, the ECM is produced by the generative cells (fibroblasts, neuroblasts, myoblasts, osteoblasts, etc.). But the energetics of the ECM (e.g. stretching of tendons, movement of muscles, elastic properties of bones, oxygenation of capillaries) affect the activities of the cells within it. Varela & Frenk refer to this as a cycle of reciprocal interaction. Such local reciprocity is also conditioned by the continuity of each local ECM with adjacent ones, and, eventually, with the ECM of the entire organism. There must be a dynamic complementarity between the overall body shape, movements of the organism, and local ECM/cell relations, and vice versa. They refer to this as a morphocycle, a continuous process of reciprocal interaction between global properties and local activities.

At any given time in the life history of an organism, its global properties (i.e. its shape and movement patterns) and its local properties (e.g. the flexibility, elasticity, or energetic continuity of a particular layer of fascia and the other 'peri-' tissues) are the culmination of its history of morphocycles. Obviously trauma of any kind sets up a series of morphocycles. Global activities and structure are inseparable from local cellular activities.

Keep in mind that all of these systems also interdigitate in important and particular ways. Figure 15.5 is a summary of these interconnections. We can view this as both a structural/energetic arrangement, for conveying tension from tissue to tissue, and as a piezoelectric solid state communication system that generates and conducts information on the activities taking place to the cells that maintain and adapt the various systems according to the ways the body is used.

Again, these fiber systems, with their obvious mechanical and architectural roles, are now recognized as important communication and metabolic systems as well. They are part of a semiconducting tensegrous vibratory continuum that allows all parts of the organism to communicate with all others. Adey (1993) refers to this as 'whispering between cells'.

Biological physics

Biologists have long suspected that living systems have evolved ways to optimally utilize all of the laws of physics and forces of nature. Some physicists

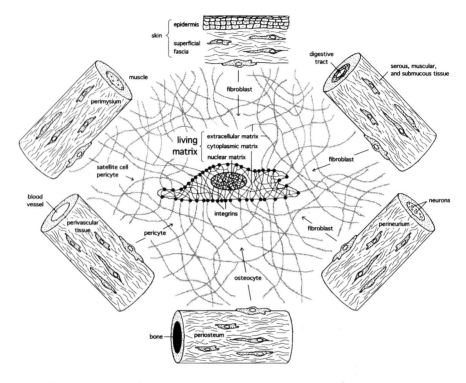

Fig. 15.5 An appreciation of the systemic interconnectedness of the living matrix system is essential to understanding the energetics of health, disease and emotional states. The tissues surrounding the digestive tract, nerves, bones, blood vessels, muscles and underlying the skin contain a sparse but active and important population of generative cells that form and continuously modify the extracellular matrix and play key roles in injury repair and defense against disease. All of these cells, and their DNA, are part of a structural, energetic and informational continuum.

have even been inspired to look for new physical concepts and laws by studying living systems (see Peliti 1991). Biological physics is a field that is likely to be very productive in the future, particularly when more physicists become aware of the high degree of crystallinity and coherence present in living systems, and the solid state properties of biological networks.

The information summarized so far leads to a simple structure–energy–communication model of living tissue that has significance for all forms of therapy. To introduce the model, we examine the physics of a helical spring. The spring is chosen because many of the key molecules in the living matrix continuum are helical: collagen, elastin, keratin, DNA, actin, and myosin (Fig. 15.6). Moreover, the spiral and the helix show up in many of the structures in the body, in the body as a whole, and in systems throughout nature (see e.g. Schwenk 1965, Stevens 1974).

Figure 15.7 shows how a wire spring converts energy from one form to another. The transformations are described with the terms used by physicists to define the different kinds of energy. We must keep in mind a fundamental conservation law of physics: energy cannot be created or destroyed, it can only be converted from one form to another.

Also keep in mind that the helical molecules in living systems are piezoelectric semiconductors. They have the capability of emitting and absorbing light and converting light energy into vibrations that can travel about within the living matrix. Because semiconductors display the transverse Hall effect, they can also respond to magnetic and biomagnetic fields.

The example of the physics of energy in a spring has a number of biological and therapeutic implications. Chapters 4 and 11 described the tensegrity model that has been used to account for energetic aspects of living systems. Figure 15.8 represents the 'tendons' of the tensegrity model as springs, each of which has the capability of absorbing and emitting the different forms of energy. As a model of living tissue, this scheme describes in a simple way how the energies used in various therapies are absorbed and conducted by the living matrix.

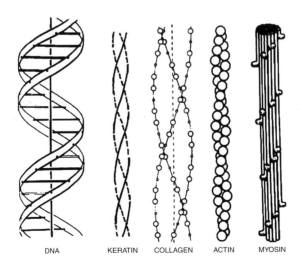

DNA   KERATIN   COLLAGEN   ACTIN   MYOSIN

Fig. 15.6 Helical molecules in the living matrix.

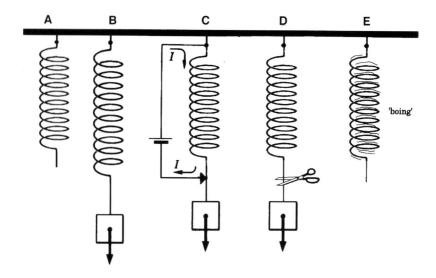

Fig. 15.7 Transformation of energy from one form to another.
A A wire spring is suspended from a solid support such as a ceiling.
B A weight is attached to the spring. The spring is stretched as the
gravitational potential energy of the weight is converted to the kinetic
energy of motion and to elastic energy in the spring. **C** A battery is
connected to the two ends of the spring, causing an electric field to
flow through the spring. The electricity generates a magnetic field that
attracts the loops of the spring toward each other, and the weight is
lifted. By lifting the weight, the spring has converted electricity to
magnetism to gravitational potential energy. **D** The attachment of the
weight is cut so the weight drops to the floor (gravitational potential
energy is converted to kinetic energy of motion). **E** The spring,
suddenly released from the tension of the weight, recoils (elastic is
converted to kinetic energy of motion) and 'boings' (elastic energy is
converted to sound).

A massage therapist touches and rubs the tissue, a herbalist applies an extract
of a plant, an acupuncturist applies a needle, magnet, electrical stimulation, or
laser beam, a shiatsu practitioner applies deep pressure, a practitioner of the
Rolf technique stretches a layer of fascia, a sound therapist vibrates the tissue,
a medical doctor uses a pulsating electromagnetic field, etc. The common
denominator in all of these approaches is a living matrix that is exquisitely
designed to absorb the information encoded in different kinds of vibratory
energy and convert it into signals that are readily transmitted through the
tensegrous semiconducting living matrix continuum.

Below we look at a vibratory property of the living matrix that is relevant to
all therapies.

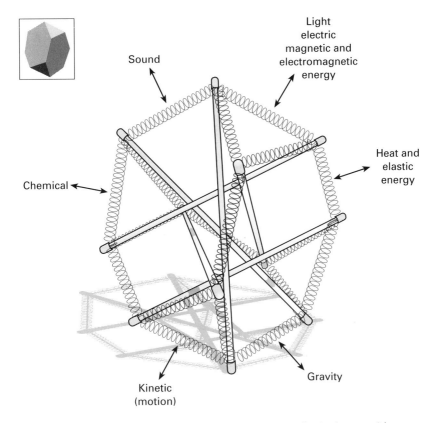

Fig. 15.8 The tensegrity model of Buckminster Fuller is drawn with the 'tendons' represented as coils. On the basis of Figure 13.7 and the discussion in the text, each of the coils has the capability of converting energy from one form to another. Because living tissue is an elastic tensegrous semiconducting continuum, any form of energy can be readily absorbed and conducted from one area to another.

Relationship of resonances to emotional states

Among the most significant of recent discoveries involving energetics is that concerning the physiological rhythms associated with certain feeling states, such as love, peace, and appreciation. The discovery has profound implications for all hands-on therapists. The research has been summarized by scientists from the Institute of HeartMath (McCraty et al 1993, Rein & McCraty 1993, Childre 1994). Particular emotional states have been correlated with measurable changes in the electrical energy spectrum of the heart.

Some of the results are shown in Figure 15.9. Heart rates are shown for an individual feeling frustration (top panel) versus appreciation (middle panel). In frustration, the heart rate varies somewhat randomly, a condition the authors refer to as incoherence. The various oscillators in the body exhibit simple harmonic or sine wave behavior of different phase, frequency, and amplitude.

Various practices that intentionally focus one's attention on the area of the heart, while invoking sincere feelings of love and appreciation, lead to a more regular variation in heart rate, a condition the authors refer to as coherence. This regular variation reflects a balance and coherence between the heart rate and the rhythms of the two branches of the autonomic nervous system, the sympathetic and parasympathetic, that regulate heart rate.

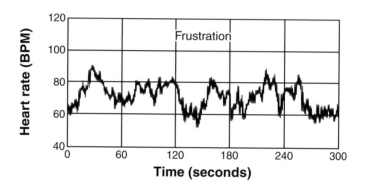

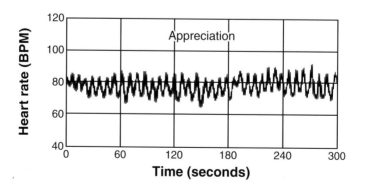

Fig. 15.9 New electrophysiological correlates associated with intentional heart focus. (From McCraty et al 1993, p. 254, fig. 1a, ISN: 1084–2209. Reproduced with kind permission of the International Society for the Study of Subtle Energies and Energy Medicine, 356 Goldco Circle, Golden, Colorado 80403. Tel: 303-425-4625.)

With appropriate intention and training, a third state can be achieved that is referred to as internal coherence. Here the variation in heart rate decreases almost to zero (lower panel). According to Childre (1994) and McCraty and colleagues (1993), this is a calm, peaceful, harmonious, and highly intuitive feeling state, in which one becomes aware of one's electrical body and of the minute currents flowing throughout. This state is associated with a coupling, or entrainment, or phase-locking of a variety of electrical and mechanical rhythms, including the heart, respiration, autonomics, and the baroreceptor feedback loop to the brain. These highly ordered physiological states, with optimum coupling of rhythms, beneficially affect the functioning of the whole body, including the brain. The reason for this follows:

Biophysics of internal coherence

A relationship between DNA and heart coherence has been suggested by work of Rein & McCraty (1993; see also Resources list at the end of this chapter). Their model involves the well-documented ability of DNA to act as a resonant antenna. The authors suggest that the DNA throughout the body both receives and transmits information encoded in the heart's electrical rhythms and in the oscillations of the DNA molecule itself.

What has been unclear about the model of Rein & McCraty (1993) is the precise mechanism by which the heart rhythms interact with DNA. The resonant properties of DNA molecules are well-documented (e.g. Pienta & Coffey 1991), as is the response of DNA to pulsing magnetic fields (e.g. Liboff et al 1984, Takahashi et al 1986). Moreover, it has recently been discovered that DNA molecules have a tendency to pack together in a crystalline array (Peterson 1997), which affects their resonance. (Crystals are widely used in radio and other electronic devices to provide precisely tuned circuits.)

A related and fascinating discovery is that the ventricle of the heart is actually formed of a single band of muscle that is wrapped in a double helix (Guasp 1980, 1987, 1995; see also Resources list at the end of this chapter). Hence the resonance Rein and colleagues suggest can be envisioned as slow oscillations of a macroscopic double helix, the heart, measured in beats per second (Fig. 15.9), resonating with the rapid oscillations of DNA, in the order of 10^{-11} to 10^{-12} per second.

A molecular explanation has emerged from consideration of the living matrix concept. The rhythmic coherences described by McCraty and colleagues (1993) can arise and propagate in part because of the piezoelectric and other solid state properties of the living matrix. The piezoelectric effect (pressure electricity) is reversible: mechanical waves generate electrical waves, and electric waves produce mechanical waves. These are called *phonons*, which are defined as electromechanical waves in a piezoelectric medium.

Hence all of the so-called acoustic or mechanical waves, such as those produced by the cranial–sacral system, the beating of the heart, the breath, muscle sounds, etc., will give rise to electromechanical waves that spread throughout the living matrix. The dual 'peri-' systems described above, and the living matrix of which they are composed, conveys these electromechanical rhythms to every nook and cranny of the body. Chemical oscillations are also entrained, via switches on the tensegrity matrix described by Ingber and colleagues (see Ch. 4). In some cases the various waves can condense into a coherent soliton wave (Oschman 1993).

One explanation of why these internal states are so beneficial is based upon new understandings of the way in which vibrating energy fields influence protein functioning. Proteins carry out all of the vital tasks in living systems, and each protein must fold in a precise way to be most effective. In an insightful chapter, 'The genetic code as language', Fröhlich (1988) suggests that oscillations set up in particular regions of the DNA create informational signals that spread throughout the body, where they energize particularly effective protein conformations.

Fröhlich's concept provides an energetic function for the large portion of the genetic material that does not code for protein amino acid sequences. Fröhlich suggests that this so-called 'nonsense', or 'selfish', or 'junk' DNA sets up signals that energize the various proteins, such as enzymes, to assume the optimal shape out of the infinite variety of configurations that are possible. The concept provides a mechanism by which the inherited DNA can regulate cell and tissue levels of complexity. The living matrix and the circulatory system are obvious candidates for the medium through which the DNA oscillations become entrained with molecules throughout the body (see also Burr and his ideas about the determination of form, Ch. 1).

A sensitive individual can begin to tune in to these phenomena by focusing on any body rhythm. The work of Childre (1994) and McCraty and colleagues (1993) focuses on the heart rhythm and then connects with other rhythms in the body. Cranial therapists begin with the cranial pulse, and often develop an awareness of other rhythms becoming entrained. The breath is another widely used entry into the rich and elegant domain of the rhythmic matrix.

The dynamic rhythmic matrix has aspects that are mechanical, electrical, magnetic, gravitational, thermal, acoustic, and photonic. Different therapeutic approaches focus on one or another of these phenomena. Because of the ability of the living matrix to extract meaningful information contained in the various kinds of energy fields, many approaches can be effective. Different individuals have different sensitivities and different skills that make it easier for them to take one route or another.

The method used by Childre (1994) and McCraty and colleagues (1993) has been termed Freeze-Frame®. Other valuable approaches to the coherent internal feeling state include the work of compassionate self-care, developed by Stephen R. Schwartz (1949–1993) (see Resources list at the end of this chapter), and the embodiment training of Will Johnson (1996).

References

Adey WR 1993 Whispering between cells: electromagnetic fields and regulatory mechanisms in tissue. Frontier Perspectives 3:21–25

Becker RO 1961 Search for evidence of axial current flow in peripheral nerves of salamander. Science 134:101–102

Becker RO 1985 Process and products involving cell modification. US Patent 4,528,265

Becker RO 1990a The machine brain and properties of the mind. Subtle Energies 1:79–87

Becker RO 1990b A technique for producing regenerative healing in humans. Frontier Perspectives 1:1–2

Becker RO 1991 Evidence for a primitive DC electrical analog system controlling brain function. Subtle Energies 2:71–88

Becker RO Selden G 1985 The body electric: electromagnetism and the foundation of life. William Morrow, New York, pp. 148

Bialek W 1984 Phonon super-radiance. Physics Letters 103A(6–7):349–352.

Bialek W 1987 Physical limits to sensation and perception. Annual Review of Biophysics and Biophysical Chemistry 16:455–478

Bonifacio R, Casagrande F, Milani M, 1984 Superradiance and superfluorescence in Josephson junction arrays. Physics Letters 101A:427–431

Burr HS 1972 Blueprint for immortality. CW Daniel, Saffron Walden, England

Childre L 1994 Freeze-Frame®. Planetary Publications, Boulder-Creek, CA

Cohen D 1967 Magnetic fields around the torso: production by electrical activity of the human heart. Science 156:652–654

Cope FW 1975 A review of the applications of solid state physics concepts to biological systems. Journal of Biological Physics 3:1–41

Cope FW 1978 Discontinuous magnetic field effects (Barkhausen noise) in nucleic acids as evidence for room temperature organic superconduction. Physiological Chemistry and Physics 10:233–246

Deecke L 1996 Planning, preparation, execution, and imagery of volitional action. Brain Research and Cognitive Brain Research 3:59–64

Deecke L, Scheid P, Kornhuber HH 1969 Distribution of readiness potential, pre-motion positivity, and motor potential of the human cerebral cortex preceding voluntary finger movements. Experimental Brain Research 7:158–168

Deecke L, Grozinger B, Kornhuber HH 1976 Voluntary finger movement in man: cerebral potentials and theory. Biological Cybernetics 23 99–119

Del Guidice E 1993 Coherence in condensed and living matter. Frontier Perspectives 3:16–20

Del Guidice E, Preparata G 1990 Superradiance: a new approach to coherent dynamical behaviors of condensed matter. Frontier Perspectives 1:16–17

Fawcett DW 1994 A Textbook of Histology, 12th edn. Chapman & Hall, New York

Feynman RP 1996 Feynman lectures on computation, ed. AJG Hey and RW Allen. Addison-Wesley, Reading, MA

Foss L 1997 Intentionality, science, and mind–body medicine: the conceptual problem. Advances: Journal of Mind–Body Health 13:70–73

Fröhlich H 1988 The genetic code as language. In: Fröhlich H (ed) Biological coherence and response to external stimuli. Springer-Verlag, Berlin, pp. 192–204

Glees P 1955 Neuroglia: morphology and function. C C Thomas, Springfield, IL

Green DE 1973 Mechanism of energy transduction in biological systems. New York Academy of Sciences Conference. Science 181:583–584

Guasp FT 1980 La estructuración macroscópica del miocardio ventricular. Revista Española de Cardiología 33:265–287

Guasp FT 1987 Macroscopical structure of the heart. (English translation of article entitled 'nuevos conceptos sobre la estructura miocárdica ventricular: estructura y mecanica del corazon) Grass Ediciones, Barcelona, Spain

Guasp FT 1995 The band-like structure of the heart unveiled by the blunt unwinding technique in practice. First Workshop of the European Working Group on Cardiac Imaging Encompasses Structure and Performance, June 9–11, 1995, Alicante, Spain

Guba F, Marechal G, Takács O 1981 Mechanism of muscle adaptation to functional requirements. Advances in Physiological Sciences. Pergamon Press, Budapest

Hamer JR 1965 Biological entrainment of the human brain by low frequency radiation. Northrop Space Laboratories, pp. 65–199

Hamer J R 1969 Effects of low level, low frequency electric fields on human time judgment. Fifth International Biometeorological Congress, Montreux, Switzerland

Johnson W 1996 Change, transformation, and the universal pattern of myofascial holding. Rolf Lines 24:2–29

Kasai T, Kawai S, Kawanishi M, Yahagi S 1997 Evidence for facilitation of motor evoked potentials (MEPs) induced by motor imagery. Brain Research 744:147–150

König 1974 ELF and VLF signal properties: physical characteristics. In: Persinger M A (ed) ELF and VLF electromagnetic field effects. Plenum Press, New York

Liboff AR, Williams T Jr, Strong DM, Wistar R Jr 1984 Time-varying magnetic fields: effect on DNA synthesis. Science 223:818–820

Little WA 1964 Possibility of synthesizing an organic superconductor. Physical Review 134:A1416–A1424

London F 1950. Superfluids, vol 1. John Wiley, New York

McCraty R, Atkinson M, Tiller W A 1993 New electrophysiological correlates associated with intentional heart focus. Subtle Energies 4(3):251–268

Mauro A, Shafiq SA, Milhorat AT 1970 Regeneration of striated muscle, and myogenesis. Excerpta Medica, Amsterdam

Meyers AW, Whelan JP, Murphy SM 1996 Cognitive behavioral strategies in athletic performance enhancement. Progress in Behavior Modification 30:137–164

Murphy M 1992 The future of the body: explorations into the further evolution of human nature. Jeremy P Tarcher/ Perigee, Los Angeles, CA, pp. 443–447

Okada Y 1983 Motor field. In: Williamson SJ, Romani G-L, Kaufman L, Modena I. (eds). An interdisciplinary approach. NATO Advanced Science Institutes Series, vol 66 section 12.7 in Biomagnetism. Plenum Press, New York, pp. 422–432

Oschman JL 1990 Bioelectromagnetic communication. BEMI Currents: the Newsletter of Bio-Electro-Magnetics Institute 2:11–14

Oschman JL 1993 Sensing solitons in soft tissues. Guild News 2:22–25

Oschman JL 1997 Connective tissue energetics, part 1: introduction to a presentation for the Stichting Opleiding Manuele Therapie, Amersfoort, The Netherlands, June 14, 1997

Oschman JL, Oschman NH 1997 Readings on the scientific basis of bodywork, energetic, and movement therapies. NORA Press, Dover, NH

Paivio A 1985 Cognitive and motivational functions of imagery in human performance. Canadian Journal of Applied Sport Science 10:22S–28S

Pauling L 1936 The diamagnetic anisotropy of aromatic molecules. Journal of Chemical Physics 4:673

Peliti L 1991 Biologically inspired physics. Proceedings of a NATO Advanced Research Workshop, September 3–13, 1990, Cargese, France. Plenum Press, New York

Peterson I 1997 Getting physical with DNA: stretching, twisting, prodding, and packing molecular strands. Science News 151:256–257

Pienta KJ Coffey DS 1991 Cellular harmonic information transfer through a tissue tensegrity-matrix system. Medical Hypotheses 34:88–95

Rein G, McCraty R 1993 Modulation of DNA by coherent heart frequencies. Proceedings of the 3rd Annual Conference of the International Society for the Study of Subtle Energies and Energy Medicine. Monterey, CA, June, 1993

Reiter R 1953 Neuere Untersuchungen zum Problem der Wetterabhängigkeit des Menschen. Archiv für Meteorologie Geophysik Bioklimatologie B4:327 (For a review of Reiter's work in English, see König HL 1974 Behavioral changes in human subjects associated with ELF electric fields. In: Persinger MA (ed) ELF and VLF electromagnetic field effects. Plenum Press, New York, pp. 81–99)

Roffey LE 1993 Why magnetic therapy works. Massage 44:3439

Roffey LE 1994 The bioelectronic basis for 'healing energies'; charge and field effects as a basis for complementary medical techniques. In: Allen MJ, Cleary SF, Sowers AE (eds) Charge and field effects in biosystems 4. Proceedings of an International Symposium held at Virginia Commonwealth University, Richmond, VA. World Scientific, Singapore, pp. 480–497

Schrödinger E 1945 What is life? The physical aspects of the living cell. Macmillan, New York

Schwenk T 1965 Sensitive Chaos: The creation of flowing forms in water and air. Rudolf Steiner Press, London

Sedlak WS 1971 Outline of biological magnetohydrodynamics. Kosmos, Series A, vol 20, Notebook 3:191–201 (An English translation of this article is available from Leane E. Roffey, Neuro-Magnetic Systems, 999 East Basse Road, Suite 180, San Antonio, TX 78209, USA. Tel: 210-824-5352)

Sedlak WS 1979 Bioelektronika 1967–1977 Institytut Wydawniczy Pax, Warszawa

Sedlak WS 1982 Bioelektronika. Proceedings of the First National Symposium on Bioelectronics, Lubin, Poland, May 14–15, 1975

Sermonti G 1995 The inadequacy of the molecular approach in biology. Frontier Perspectives 4:31–34

Seto A, Kusaka C, Nakazato S, Hang W, Sato T, Hisamitsu T, Takeshige C 1992 Detection of extraordinary large bio-magnetic field strength from human hand. Acupuncture and Electrotherapeutics Research International Journal 17; 75–94

Stent G 1972 Prematurity and uniqueness in scientific discovery. Scientific American 277:84–93

Stevens PS 1974 Patterns in nature. Little Brown, Boston, MA

Suinn RM 1985 Imagery rehearsal: application to performance enhancement. Behavior Therapist 8:155–159

Takahashi K, Kaneko I, Date M, Fukada E 1986 Effect of pulsing electromagnetic fields on DNA synthesis in mammalian cells in culture. Experientia 42:185–186

Varela FJ, Frenk S 1987 The organ of form: towards a theory of biological shape. Journal of Social and Biological Structures 10:73–83

Warner L, McNeill ME 1988 Mental imagery and its potential for physical therapy. Physical Therapy 68:516–521

Williamson SJ, Kaufman L 1981 Biomagnetism. Journal of Magnetism and Magnetic Materials 22:129–201

Wolf AA 1976 Experimental evidence for high-temperature organic fractional superconduction in cholates. Physiological Chemistry and Physics 8:495–518

Wolf AA, Halpern EH 1976 Experimental high temperature organic superconductivity in the cholates: a summation of results. Physiological Chemistry and Physics 8:31–36

Wolf AA, Halpern EH, Sherman J 1976 Diamagnetic levitation in the fractionally superconducting bile cholates. Physiological Chemistry and Physics 8:135–142

Wu C 1997 A magnet for a future atom smasher. Science News 151(31 May):340

Zimmerman J 1985 New technologies detect effects of healing hands. Brain/Mind Bulletin 10:2

Resources

A plastic model depicting the double spiral arrangement of the musculature in the human heart (discovered by Guasp) is available from Merck, Sharp & Dohme de España, S.A., Josef Valcárcel 38, 27028 Madrid, Spain

The articles on the modulation of DNA by coherent heart frequencies (by Rein & McCraty) and related articles are available from the Institute of HeartMath, PO Box 1436, 14700 West Park Avenue, Boulder Creek, CA 95006, USA. Tel: 408–338–8700. Fax: 408-338-9861

Schwartz SR Various books and cassettes available from Compassionate Self-Care Publications, PO Box 28214, Seattle, WA 98118-8214, USA. Tel: 206-725-6920

16 Energy circles

Demonstrating the flow of energy in groups

Fifteen years of multidisciplinary research and teaching have provided the background for this book (Oschman & Oschman 1997). Workshops given at many different locations have led to a method for demonstrating the flow of energy in groups. The energy circle encompasses many of the concepts presented in this book. It is based primarily on the linking of biological rhythms in a group of people, and using imagery and movement techniques to increase the awareness of energy flows through the hands.

We begin by forming the group into a circle. To achieve a more relaxed state, everyone is asked to smile vigorously and ridiculously. This is not only amusing, but it affects everyone's emotional state. The basis for this is the well-documented but little-known relationship between facial muscle tension, cerebral blood flow and subjective feelings (Zajonc 1985).

To entrain the breath, participants are instructed to inhale deeply together and exhale through their mouths vigorously enough to push their cheeks outward.

To intentionally focus attention on the area of the heart, participants place their fingers on their breast bones, inhale deeply and hum with lips closed as loud as they can. With a few repetitions of this exercise, the sound vibrations can be felt in the heart area and the tone becomes more deep and resonant. Many feel a tingling in their cheeks.

Any pulsing signal, sound, light, electric, or magnetic can entrain brain waves (see Ch. 5). We use a technique called the bell breath. A pair of Tibetan bells is struck together to produce a soothing tone. The author has analyzed the frequency spectrum of these bells, individually and together. Both bells have a fundamental tone of about 2500 Hz. Each bell has a different vibrato frequency, one at 9 Hz and the other at 26 Hz (Fig. 16.1). These frequencies are ideal to entrain the brain waves. The 9 Hz signal is in the alpha range. For the

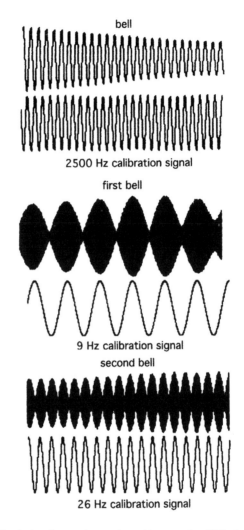

Fig. 16.1 Analysis of sounds produced by a pair of Tibetan bells. The fundamental tone of each bell is 2500 Hz. One bell has a vibrato of about 9 Hz, while the other is about 26 Hz. The tones were analyzed with a Macintosh computer, using MacRecorder and SoundEdit™ software.

bell breath, the group is asked to hold hands, close eyes and take a deep breath when they hear the tone. The reason for closing the eyes is that it is easier to enter alpha with the eyes closed (Fig. 2.5).

After several bell breaths, we suggest the possibility of entraining heart rhythms. The heart is the strongest source of electricity in the body, and the field can be detected anywhere on the skin surface. Because sweat is a good conductor, components of the heart electricity spread from person to person in the circle. It is possible, but unlikely that all of the group's fundamental heart rhythms will entrain. Instead, an effort is made to entrain the higher frequency components of the electrocardiogram, discussed in the context of the work of McCraty and colleagues (Ch. 15).

To accomplish this, participants are asked to visualize a time in their lives when they were exceptionally happy, and take several more bell breaths. The aim is to produce internal coherence as described by McCraty and colleagues, including the higher frequency components of the electrocardiogram.

The next process is designed to bring awareness of the entrained rhythms to the hands. Participants are asked to open their eyes, drop their hands to their sides, shake their hands vigorously and then rub them together. Next they place their palms and fingers together, almost but not quite touching, and move their hands closer and farther away, to see if they detect a sensation of energy. Some feel this effect as a magnet-like sensation and others feel warmth.

To enhance the sensation, participants are asked to perform a 'micro-movement'. This is a movement that is enormously stretched out over time. The participants are asked to bring their hands together, but to take a week to do it. This process heightens the kinesthetic awareness of the hands, without producing actual movement. As described in the previous chapter, the process sets up the readiness and feedback fields, without the motor fields that would trigger actual movement.

Finally, everyone turns 90° to the right and places their hands next to but not touching the back of the person in front of them. They close their eyes and do several bell breaths. A palpable 'energy' flows counterclockwise around the circle.

At this point a massage table is brought into the circle. A volunteer with a physical or emotional difficulty, or a skeptic, is asked to lie on the table, and a simple circuit is created as shown in Figure 16.2. At one end of the circle, a person holds their hands on or near the subject's head, and at the other end someone holds their hands on or near the subject's feet. Several more bell breaths enhance the flow of energy through the group and the subject. At this point, a 'hands-on' or energetic therapist can perform a technique on the subject.

The energy circles have yielded many fascinating and unexpected results. Individuals with physical problems, such as sore joints, often feel a sensation of warmth in the affected area and subsequent lessening of their problems.

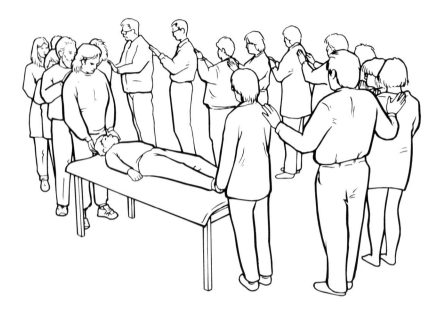

Fig. 16.2   An energy circle.

Deeply held emotional traumas sometimes resolve spontaneously. One partici-pant found that she no longer needed her hearing aid. Others simply report that they have acquired an ability to sense energy fields with their hands. Therapists report greater ease and sensitivity in performing their techniques.

The energy circle is a 'laboratory' in which we can simultaneously explore the great discoveries of biology and bodywork. One unifying hypothesis is that the essence that nourishes the living matrix, and that is lacking in those places of disorder or pain, is information. Living systems probably utilize all forms of energy to convey information into every corner of the body. A part of the hypothesis is that this kind of nourishment can be projected from the tips of the fingers. When this happens, one has an experience of the composite flow of the various kinds of biological energy. Once supplied in the pure form that can come only from another organism, the information directs the repair systems of the body to repair themselves. The side-effects are always beneficial, sometimes magnificent.

References

Oschman JL, Oschman NH 1997 Readings on the scientific basis of bodywork, movement, and energetic therapies. NORA Press, Dover, NH

Zajonc RB Emotion and facial efference: a theory reclaimed. Science 228: 15–21

Afterword: clarity and consensus emerge from the tangle of controversy and confusion

If the history of science has a lesson for us, it is that 'consensus among the experts' can undergo rapid change. For example:

◈ A few decades ago the suggestion that organisms have energy fields around them, and that these fields can produce meaningful interactions between organisms, had little scientific credibility.

◈ The repeated observation of naturalists that geophysical and celestial rhythms influence plant and animal behavior seemed utterly preposterous to all but a few scientists.

◈ Healing with natural or artificial energy fields had the same scientific acceptance as voodoo, levitation, and UFOs.

◈ When concern arose about possible health effects of exposure to electromagnetic fields from appliances and other technologies, many experts stated that these energies are far too weak to have any biological effects.

Intense research into these subjects has led to a complete reversal of opinion. Key to these developments have been collaborations between the physical, biological, and molecular sciences. Here is the current opinion of a number of the experts:

> [There is]...a growing scientific consensus on the cell and molecular biology mediating interactions with environmental electromagnetic fields. Beyond the chemistry of molecules that form the exquisite fabric of living tissues, we now discern a new frontier in biological organization...based on physical processes at the atomic level, rather than in chemical reactions between biomolecules... these physical processes may powerfully regulate the products of biochemical reactions. (Adey 1996)

> In the last decade, evidence has rapidly accumulated that supports the hypothesis that exposure to low energy nonionizing radiation can induce and/ or modulate events within biological tissues. (Goodman & Henderson 1987)

249

There is now convincing evidence from a large number of laboratories, that exposure to extremely low frequency (ELF) magnetic and electric fields produces biological responses in animals. (Anderson 1996)

...there is general agreement that exogenous electric and electromagnetic fields influence and modulate the properties of biological systems. (Blank & Findl 1987)

... many of the leading researchers in the field of bioelectrochemistry / biomagnetics agree that exogenous fields modify cellular calcium ion transport. (Findl 1987)

Enzymatic processes themselves are field-sensitive. (Westerhoff et al 1987)

...weak electric fields can change the probability that molecules of the reacting materials will encounter each other... (Barnes 1996)

By amplification we are referring to a situation in which a tiny field, far too weak to power any cellular activity, triggers a change at the regulatory level which then leads to a substantial physiological response that is carried out using the energy of cell metabolism. (Pilla et al 1987)

Recent progress in the application of electromagnetic energy has revolutionized many areas of medicine. (Chandos et al 1996)

Complementing the literature cited above is a detailed and thoughtful analysis of the biophysical and medical significance of the new developments (Bistolfi 1991).

Scientific consensus has gone from a certainty that weak environmental energies can have no influence on living systems to agreement that such influences are extremely important and deserving of intense study to determine the precise mechanisms involved.

Collectively, the discoveries of modern researchers tell a story of biological sensitivity that coincides with the daily experiences of energy therapists ranging from medical doctors using PEMF techniques to acupuncturists to polarity therapists, Reiki practitioners, herbalists, aromatherapists and so on. The new concepts do not require us to abandon our sophisticated understandings of physiology, biochemistry or molecular biology. Instead, they extend our picture of living processes, and of healing, to finer levels of structure and function. Our definition of living matter is being expanded to incorporate the physics and chemistry of the solid state, including semiconduction, quantum mechanics, liquid crystals, and biological coherence (see for example Ho 1998, Ho et al 1994).

A few long cherished assumptions have proven inadequate. For many years biologists and physicists agreed that fields can only have effects if the energy level is sufficient to cause heating or ionization of the tissues. The threshold for all biological stimuli was assumed to be set by intrinsic physical factors: atomic collisions (heat) and noise. We now know that tiny amounts of energy at the appropriate frequency can produce profound biological effects, without heating or ionizing tissues, even in the presence of much higher levels of noise.

We are learning that cells maintain their organized society by 'whispering together' in a faint and private language (Adey 1996). The 'whispers' travel as both chemical and electromagnetic messages. Learning the electromagnetic codes used in these whispers has become a new and important focus for researchers, and obviously has enormous clinical importance. We will soon know the electromagnetic languages of all of the cells in the body, including those of bacteria and tumor cells. In the past, we thought the words of the 'language of life' were nerve impulses and molecules, but we now see that there is a deeper layer of communication underlying these familiar processes. Beneath the relatively slow moving action potentials and billiard ball interactions of molecules lies a much faster and subtle realm of interactions. This dimension is subatomic, energetic, electromagnetic and wave-like in character. The chemical messenger ultimately transfers its information electromagnetically. Hence the electromagnetic code is actually primary. Nerve impulses and chemical messengers are contained within the individual whereas energy fields radiate indefinitely into space and therefore affect others who are nearby. For millennia, energy therapists have had a practical appreciation of these phenomena, which are finally open to scientific research.

The electromagnetic language has two aspects, frequency and intensity. After much confusion, extensive laboratory research is confirming what the homeopathic physician or aromatherapist has known for a long time: when it comes to triggering healing responses, 'small is powerful', or 'less is more'. The search for an appropriate essence is in fact a search for compounds with the correct molecular emission spectrum to provide benefit for a particular ailment in a particular patient at a particular time.

In *Molecules of Emotion*, Candace Pert (1997) speculates on how energy healers may use their own energy fields to trigger receptors in the bodies of their patients. She calls for basic research into this promising area. Her careful research on neuropeptides can be integrated with the emerging understandings of electromagnetics to give us a much clearer picture of the human body in health and disease, and the biophysics of emotions.

An important example of the progress being made is found in Chapter 9, where we discussed system-wide regulations and separated out a single physiological control loop from the web of balance and coordination processes in the body (see Fig. 9.8). This was described as a cascade of chemical reactions accompanied by a cascade of electronic and electromagnetic interactions. This has become a vigorous and productive area of research, for all living processes are ultimately carried out by cells and by the molecules and by the energy fields they produce. We are learning precisely which steps in the cellular/molecular/electromagnetic cascade are particularly sensitive to exogenous energy fields and which ones are not. We are also discovering how minute signals from the environment are amplified to produce large cellular effects. The significance of cellular amplification was recognized by the 1994 Nobel Prize in Physiology or Medicine (Gilman 1997).

In essence, we are discovering the molecular and electromagnetic basis for cybernetics. This term was coined by Norbert Wiener (1948), who defined it as the science of communication and control. Cybernetics is derived from the Greek word *kybernetes*, meaning helmsman. The helmsman can change the course of a huge vessel virtually effortlessly by applying a small adjustment to the tiller. Likewise, a small energy field applied at the appropriate place and time can shift the course of an organism.

Figure A-1 summarizes our current understanding of the signaling cascade and the portions that have been identified as sensitive to electromagnetic fields. Receptors on the cell surface are the primary sites of action of low frequency electromagnetic fields. It is at the receptor that cellular responses are triggered by hormones, growth factors, neurotransmitters, taste and smell molecules, pheromones, light and a variety of other electromagnetic signals. Membrane proteins closely associated with receptors, such as adenylate cyclases and G proteins, couple a single molecular event at the cell surface to the influx of a huge number of calcium ions. Calcium ions entering the cell activate a variety of enzyme molecules. The enzymes, in turn, are catalysts, greatly accelerating biochemical processes. Catalysts are not consumed by reactions. Hence the enzymes can act again and again until calcium levels drop back to pre-stimulation levels.

The frequency of the stimulus is crucial. For example, separate studies of lymphocytes stimulated with a mitogen showed that a weak 3 Hz pulsed magnetic field sharply *reduced* calcium influx, while a 60 Hz signal, under identical conditions *increased* calcium influx (see Adey 1996 for references).

New research is revealing how free radicals, including nitric oxide, are involved in the coupling of electromagnetic fields to chemical events in the signal cascade. Again, the medical importance of this research has been recognized by a Nobel Prize (Furchgott et al 1998). Because intermediates in enzymatic reactions can be electrically charged free radicals, magnetic

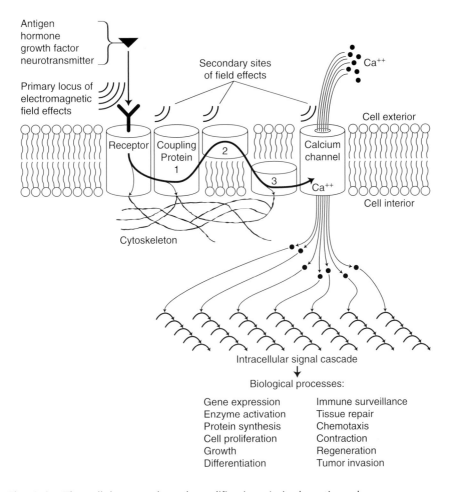

Fig. A-1 The cellular cascade and amplification. A single antigen, hormone, pheromone, growth factor, or smell or taste or neurotransmitter molecule, or a single photon of electromagnetic energy, can produce a cascade of intracellular signals that initiate, accelerate, or inhibit biological processes. This is possible because of enormous amplification – a single molecular event at the cell surface can trigger a huge influx of calcium ions, each of which can activate an enzyme. The enzymes, in turn, act as catalysts, greatly accelerating biochemical processes. The enzymes are not consumed by these reactions, and can therefore act repeatedly. Some of the reactions are sensitive to electromagnetic fields, some are not, and others have not yet been tested. Some frequencies enhance calcium entry, others diminish it. Steps in the cascade involving free radical formation are likely targets of magnetic fields. Some of the products of the cascade are returned back to the cell surface and into the surrounding extracellular space. Molecular events within cells set up electronic, photonic, and electromechanical waves (phonons) that propagate as solitons through the cellular and extracellular matrix. These feedbacks enable cells and tissues to form a functionally organized society. The cells whisper to each other in a faint and private language. They can 'tune into' each other over long ranges.

fields can cause the reactants to twist or drift during the very short time intervals when they are interacting. Such phenomena are being examined in great detail using 'femtochemistry,' in which ultra-short flashes of laser light provide a sort of 'slow motion' analysis of the steps in chemical reactions. The ability to make such precise measurements on chemical reactions is so important that the methods have been recognized by the Nobel Committee (Zewail 1999).

The inset for Figure 9.8 showed the way the various elements of the signal cascade absorb and emit electromagnetic signals as they carry out their roles. Benveniste (1998) has emphasized these interactions in his model (see Fig. 14.1).

In accord with Benveniste's model, the cellular cascades we know the most about are triggered by electromagnetic fields rather than molecular signals. The most carefully studied systems are the photoreceptors in the retina of the eye, and the chloroplast that extracts energy from sunlight. Stryer (1987) has reviewed the details of photoreception, and presented a model showing that the cellular response to various hormones is virtually identical to the response to an electromagnetic field (light). Stryer's illustration is conceptually identical to Benveniste's.

As usual, these important new ideas are greeted with resistance and skepticism. For example, Benveniste has now received a second 'Ig Nobel' prize by the editor of something called *The Annals of Improbable Research*. In contention is Benveniste's work showing that a solution's biological activity can be digitally recorded, stored on a computer hard drive, sent over the Internet as an attached document, and transferred to a water sample at the receiving end (Nadls 1998). Since Benveniste's findings are based on a simple logic and do not violate any accepted principles, their 'improbability' seems to derive from the prejudices and irrational resistance of his detractors. The study of electromagnetism in living systems continues to be threatening to some. James Randi, a magician with no scientific credibility or credentials, does not like Benveniste's work, and his disparaging remarks have been published in *Nature*. Now, *Nature* is usually regarded as a respectable and discriminating scientific journal. Unfortunately the magazine has published Randi's comments even though they contain no logical arguments or evidence of any kind for rejecting Benveniste's discoveries.

In fact, to deny direct electromagnetic interactions with living molecules would be to deny the fundamental reaction upon which all life depends, namely the absorption of sunlight by green plants. The mechanisms involved are no more mysterious than is spectroscopy, the primary method by which scientists study the structure of atoms and molecules.

The energy circle described in Chapter 16 can provide a fascinating experience of the phenomenon of direct electromagnetic interactions of the type described by Benveniste. During a recent workshop at Misty Meadows Herbal Center in Lee, New Hampshire, an herbal remedy, hawthorn, was introduced into the energy circle. An intact hawthorn branch was placed on a table and two of the participants in the circle placed their hands over it, without touching. A number of the people in the circle felt an immediate calming or tingling effect. That this is not the result of suggestion was demonstrated in a subsequent work-shop in England in which the presence of the hawthorn in the energy circle led to an immediate sensation of the smell of the plant in a person who had been unable to smell anything for 20 years because of an injury that had destroyed her olfactory epithelium. Simultaneously another participant experienced the odor of the plant even though she had a cold and had not been able to smell anything for several days. The simple explanation for these unanticipated phenomena is that the electromagnetic signature of the plant can quickly enter the group's energy field and communicate its effects. As Benveniste has suggested, molecules can 'tune into' each other over long ranges.

Woodhouse (1996) gives a well-reasoned summary of the process in which new reliable data and ideas are first resisted and then become incorporated into contemporary thought. His description is particularly relevant to concepts related to energy medicine, which have such a long history of confusion and controversy. We cannot escape this history, we can only become mindful of the countless and subtle ways the past affects our attitudes. Many of the observations of energy therapists down through the ages, observations that science has previously found unacceptable, are being validated and explained by researchers from around the world. A repeating cycle in medical research is initial rejection followed by eventual appreciation for the pioneers who have made insightful and important discoveries, often in a hostile climate.

For centuries, concepts of 'life force' and 'healing energy' have been at the center of one of the most bitter and acrimonious debates in the history of science. The discussions have been saturated with confusion, controversy, antagonism, dogmas, and fear. The idea that our physiology and our personal lives can be affected by invisible forces outside of us, or by events at a great distance, has been unacceptable or uncomfortable for many:

> There is nothing that man fears more than the touch of the unknown. He wants to see what is reaching towards him, and to be able to recognize or at least classify it. (Canetti 1962)

To realize the inestimable promise of electromagnetic medicine, we must overcome the legacy of past dogmas and intolerances, and our fears of invisible forces. How rapidly this takes place depends significantly on each of us, and on our individual capacity to look within ourselves, our willingness to explore the ways our ideas, attitudes, and experiences of energy have been shaped by what we have been taught. Certainly, for a culture that has become accustomed to having large numbers of tasks handled by invisible currents flowing through chips in computers, and its television sets adjusted by invisible radiation from remote control devices, it is not too frightening to look at the ways our bodies are regulated and coordinated by invisible energies.

As an example, I was taught that Franz Anton Mesmer's concepts of 'animal magnetism' had been thoroughly discredited in 1784 by a distinguished Royal Commission in France. This was not, however, the end of Mesmer's legacy. While he was alive, Mesmer's personal life and eccentricities were the subject of much rumor. Regardless of the truth of these stories, what happened during the 19th century is quite revealing and relevant to our own times (Winter 1998).

The trance state that Mesmer initiated, by interacting with a person's 'magnetic fluids', became immensely fashionable in Victorian England during the 1830s through the 1860s and beyond. Eventually mesmerism came to be spelled with a small 'm', to distinguish its hypnotic aspects from the concept of 'magnetic fluids', which many found unacceptable. Itinerant lecturers traveled the English countryside, demonstrating their 'mesmeric' powers in public shows and private sèances. 'Altered states' were produced, during which one's movements and speech could be controlled by the hypnotist. Mesmerism spread throughout England, Ireland, the Highlands of Scotland, and the Empire. The public became fascinated with vital powers, spirits, phrenologists, mediums, and psychic researchers and experimenters of all kinds. Established scientists, doctors, and other professionals became embroiled in discussions of the meaning of the mesmeric trance state.

James Esdaile MD took mesmerism to India. Although he was initially highly skeptical and suspicious, Esdaile documented countless medical successes among the people of Bengal, including painless surgical operations performed by surgeons who were also highly skeptical of mesmerism (Esdaile 1846). The preface to Esdaile's book, written by his brother David, prophetically pointed out the potential of mesmerism for evil as well as good: 'How foolish in people to expose themselves to the machinations of the wicked, by treating mesmerism as a fraud or a delusion.'

The phenomenon of the mesmeric trance led to great debates over what was really happening and what it meant. The discussions reached every level of society, and influenced the evolution of psychological and scientific discourses as we know them today. The discussions brought up the question of who had the authority to determine the validity of any scientific or medical phenomenon. Eventually there emerged a new and previously nonexistent class of beings called 'professional scientists'. These 'experts' were empowered to derogate a particular phenomenon as marginal or fringe. The lay public was educated to suspend logical analysis in favor of the suggestions of those in authority. Concepts of mass consensus and agreement were redefined. While the lofty goal was the protection of society from quacks and charlatans, the power of authority could also be misused by vested interests to withhold important discoveries. Scientific and medical progress has suffered from this subtle form of attitude control, which has prevented mainstream exploration of valuable insights about energetics that could probably have saved countless lives.

After the enthusiastic reception in Victorian Britain, concepts of animal magnetism and mesmerism gradually passed out of mainstream medical lore and public exploration. This did not happen because of scientific breakthroughs or because the public became less gullible or because mesmerism was exposed as fraudulent. Instead, mesmerism was absorbed into other practices, particularly psychology and psychoanalysis. The areas most closely relevant to mesmerism, physiology and physics, became laboratory sciences. The phenomenon of hypnosis revealed the existence of the subconscious, and led to the subsequent explorations of Freud, Jung, and their followers.

Paradoxically, mesmerism stimulated great interest and debate about fundamental biological questions, but there was little progress in resolving them. This happened in part because biology followed the model of physics: if a phenomenon is difficult to measure or does not fit into any of the emerging disciplines, it is excluded from investigation. Mesmerism brought up profoundly important questions of the nature of the mind, but these very questions were eventually disqualified as legitimate fields for scientific research (Winter 1998). The taboo against scientific research into consciousness continued until relatively recently. Cognitive scientists and neuroscientists ignored consciousness because the problem was considered to be too 'philosophical' or too 'inaccessible' for laboratory investigation (Ingalls 1995).

This long-standing impasse was decisively hurdled in the early 1990s, when Nobel Laureate Francis Crick began to openly discuss the scientific basis of consciousness. Crick pointed out that timidity toward the study of consciousness is completely ridiculous. Mental events, he said, could be explained by the firing of large sets of neurons (see Crick & Koch 1992). Logical, testable, verifiable, and falsifiable hypotheses about consciousness can and should be generated. Eminent scientists such as Roger Penrose and Gerald Edelman agreed, and scientific books and journal articles on consciousness began to appear.

I do not agree with Crick that consciousness arises entirely as a result of the firings of neurons. Real progress in the study of consciousness will not occur until the somatic and energetic aspects are brought into consideration. For example, Charman (1997) logically views what we refer to as 'mind' in terms of a brain-generated neuromagnetic field. To paraphrase: when the mosaic of neurons resonates at preferred frequencies, so will their associated microfields. These will interact with each other to form a complex, neuromagnetic whole that permeates through the magnetically 'transparent' physical structure of the brain as if it was not there.

Max Planck long ago saw 'mind' at a finer level: 'We must assume behind this force [in the atom] the existence of a conscious and intelligent mind. This mind is the matrix of all matter.' (Network 1999). And Pearson (1997) went even further, to suggest that mind arises at a sub-quantum level of reality, which is 'structured like a neural network'. Add to these fascinating concepts of 'mind' the biomagnetic fields of the organs and peripheral neurons, semi-conduction through the cellular and subcellular structures associated with them, and the electromagnetic signatures of all of the vibrating molecules within the cells and tissues, and we begin to see a dynamic picture of the energetic body as a whole. What we refer to as 'mind' and 'consciousness' may encompass the totality of communications and regulations in the body, the electromagnetic signatures of countless molecules and atoms, and the energy fields they entail. The emergence of a discipline of psychoneuroimmunology attests to the inter-connectedness of conscious and unconscious physiological events in all of the systems in the body. Emerging concepts of consciousness have profound therapeutic implications (see Ch. 8).

Another valuable perspective on the quest to understand life and healing emerges from study of Mesmer's original writings, faithfully translated by Bloch (1980). Here Mesmer can be seen, at least in the early part of his career, as a careful scientist, striving to account for his discoveries in terms of the new and popular physical science of Isaac Newton, but without the benefit of the subsequent discoveries of Galvani, Volta, Faraday, Oersted, Nernst, and Maxwell, who later described the relations between electricity, magnetism, and electromagnetism. The fact that Mesmer became more and more eccentric in his later years can be used as a reason to dismiss his accomplishments, but, as we have seen, the way his work was developed after his death is far more significant.

Mesmer's labours to describe the physics of the 'magnetic fluids' is comparable to that of present day pioneers in energy medicine, who strive to reconcile their observations with relativity theory, quantum mechanics, and the emerging post-modern physics, so that they can explain their therapies in ways that are both comprehensible to their patients and logically consistent with modern science (e.g. Wilson 1999).

In presenting workshops on energetics, I have chosen an approach that combines the intellectual aspects with an experience of group energy flow. Chapter 16 describes the energy circles, which have become a 'laboratory' for the exploration of energy field interactions. Energy circles are an ancient tradition, used in many cultures for the purposes of healing or spiritual initiation. I am mindful of the sensational and controversial history of mesmerism, and the importance of maintaining an objective atmosphere in any group exploration. As a scientist, I have come to use the circles as a systematic study of the interaction of group consciousness, heart focus, group intention, and the physiology of healing.

Steps are taken to prevent the energy circle from becoming a theatrical or charismatic performance rather than an objective process. The experiment begins with arranging the participants into a 'circuit'. The presenter then steps back and everyone watches and senses what happens. If there is to be a single proximate 'source' of the 'healing energy' or intention, that person is not the presenter, but is chosen more or less randomly from the group.

In many workshops, we begin by showing the participants how to focus on the sensations in their hands. (The process is described in Ch. 16.) We then select someone from the group who has an ailment that has been difficult to treat. They do not reveal the details of their problem to the group. The subject lies on a treatment table. The participants then file past silently, using their hands to scan the energy field from head to foot. When everyone has made their assessment of the 'patient' we compare notes. Inevitably a large percentage of the participants have located the subject's physical ailment, and, in some cases, the exact nature of the problem, without any prior knowledge on the part of anyone in the room. Moreover, subjects often report feeling profound relief of symptoms as the group is performing its energetic scan.

Today the entire subject of magnetic fluids and mesmerism comes round, full circle, to where it began, with modern inquiries into precisely how magnetic and electromagnetic fields interact with the systems that control the body's defense and repair systems, and that keep cells from dividing uncontrollably (see, for example, the essays in the symposium edited by Ueno 1996). The primary motivation for current scientific research does not come from an interest in complementary medicine. Instead, it comes from independent lines of investigation conducted by different groups of researchers over the past 20 years or so. Because of the ways we compartmentalize knowledge, most of the scientists involved did not know how much their work was being validated by the others, nor did they realize they were laying a scientific foundation for complementary energy therapies.

Because of the ways science has been done in the past, and the history of confusion about energy, there will be some who do not think this book should have been written. My goal of connecting scientific information with complementary therapies will be viewed by some as an unacceptable endeavor. However, the unavoidable reality is that new vistas are opening up as science and complementary medicine learn how to talk to each other. Energy is a major topic in this conversation, for much is known about energetics from these perspectives that have been kept separate for reasons that no longer serve us. A major force in this exploration is the public's justifiable insistence that there be a careful and thoughtful exploration of popular and successful therapeutic strategies that have traditionally been isolated from biomedical research, practice, and teaching.

Each chapter of this book represents a major piece of the puzzle that will have its own evolution as new data and conceptual breakthroughs emerge. I have no illusion that any part of this book contains the last word on any of these subjects. This is, of course, a 'work in progress'. Each day, each visit to the library, each chat with a colleague, and each question from a student brings in a new piece of the puzzle, a new perspective.

For example, as these final words were being written, André K. Geim and his colleagues at the University of Nijmegen, in the Netherlands, showed that the water, proteins, and organic molecules in human fingers can develop magnetic properties in an applied magnetic field (this is called diamagnetism) (Geim et al 1999). The effect is strong enough to enable a pair of well-placed fingers to stabilize a magnet, as shown in Figure A-2. The Nijmegen group had previously demonstrated that the forces from living tissues were strong enough to levitate entire plants and animals, such as frogs, in a magnetic field (Berry & Geim 1997). These new discoveries are a dramatic indication of remarkable and unexpected properties possessed by living tissues.

Paradoxically, while scientists were determining that tissues can extract meaningful signals from much higher levels of electromagnetic 'noise', engineers were developing sophisticated sensing devices with similar attributes. Many of these devices have been sent, at great expense, about as far away from humans as possible, to the outer edges of the solar system, where they record the properties of the interstellar wind and other distant celestial phenomena. Why have we not turned these elegant sensors toward ourselves, to explore the kinds of energies all of us can emit? Research of this kind is of profound medical importance.

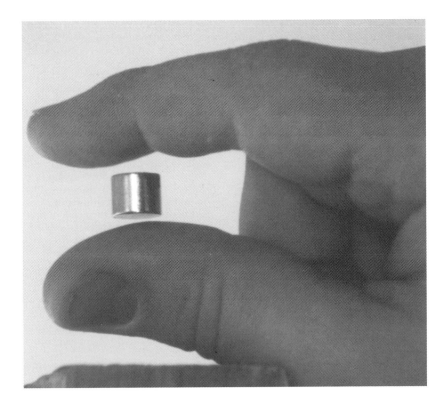

Fig. A-2 Fingertip levitation. Water, proteins, and organic molecules in human fingers can develop magnetic properties in an applied magnetic field (this is called diamagnetism). The effect is strong enough to enable a pair of well-placed fingers to stabilize a magnet. A powerful electromagnet is located 2.5 meters above the fingers. (Reproduced by kind permission of A.K. Geim, High Field Magnet Laboratory, University of Nijmegen, The Netherlands.)

References

Adey, WR 1996 A growing scientific consensus on the cell and molecular biology mediating interactions with environmental electromagnetic fields. In: Ueno S (ed) Biological effects of magnetic and electromagnetic fields. Plenum Press, New York, ch. 4, pp. 45–62

Anderson LE 1996 Investigation of exposure to extremely low frequency (ELF) magnetic and electric fields: status of laboratory animal studies. In: Ueno S (ed) Biological effects of magnetic and electromagnetic fields. Plenum Press, New York, ch. 9, pp. 131–138

Barnes FS 1996 The effects of ELF on chemical reaction rates in biological systems. In: Ueno S (ed) Biological effects of magnetic and electromagnetic fields. Plenum Press, New York, ch. 3, pp. 37–44

Benveniste J 1998 From 'water memory effects' to 'digital biology'. On the web at: http://www.digibio.com/

Berry MV, Geim AK 1997 Of flying frogs and levitrons. European Journal of Physics 18:307–313

Bistolfi F 1991 Biostructures and radiation order disorder. Edizioni Minerva Medica, Turin

Blank M, Findl E 1987 Preface to Mechanistic approaches to interactions of electric and electromagnetic fields with living systems. Plenum Press, New York

Bloch G 1980 Mesmerism. A translation of the original scientific and medical writings of FA Mesmer. William Kaufman, Inc., Los Altos, California

Canetti E 1962 Crowds and Power. Translated by Carol Stewart from the 1960 book, Masse und Macht, The Noonday Press, New York

Chandos B, Khan A, Lai H, Lin JC 1996 The application of electromagnetic energy to the treatment of neurological and psychiatric diseases. In: Ueno S (ed) Biological effects of magnetic and electromagnetic fields. Plenum Press, New York, ch. 12, pp. 161–170

Charman RA 1997 The field substance of mind: a hypothesis. Network 63:11–13.

Crick F, Koch C 1992 The problem of consciousness. Scientific American 266(3):153–159

Esdaile J 1846 Mesmerism in India and its practical application in surgery and medicine. Longman, Brown, Green, and Longmans, London, reprinted in 1976 as a classic in psychiatry by Arno Press, New York

Findl E 1987 Membrane transduction of low energy level fields and the Ca++ hypothesis. In: Blank M, Findl E (eds) Mechanistic approaches to interactions of electric and electromagnetic fields with living systems. Plenum Press, New York, pp. 15–38

Furchgott RF, Ignarro KH, Murad F 1998 Nitric oxide as a signaling molecule in the cardiovascular system. Nobel Prize in Physiology or Medicine, Karolinska Institutet.

Geim AK, Simon MD, Boamfa MI, Heflinger LO 1999 Magnet levitation at your fingertips. Nature 400:323–324

Gilman AG 1997 G proteins and regulation of adenylyl cyclase. Nobel Lecture presented December 8 1994. In: Ringertz N (ed) Nobel Lectures Physiology or Medicine, 1991–1995. World Scientific, Singapore, pp. 182–212

Goodman R Henderson AS 1987 Patterns of transcription and translation in cells exposed to EM fields: a review. In: Blank M, Findl E (eds) Mechanistic approaches to interactions of electric and electromagnetic fields with living systems. Plenum Press, New York, pp. 217–230

Ho M-W 1998 The rainbow and the worm: the physics of organisms, 2nd edn. Singapore, River Edge, New Jersey

Ho M-W, Popp F-A, Warnke U (eds) 1994 Bioelectrodynamics and biocommunication. World Scientific, Singapore, pp. 81–107

Ingalls H 1995 Consciousness as a valid subject for scientific investigation. Recent advances in brain research have stimulated widespread interest throughout the scientific community in the nature of consciousness, lending new respectability to the subject. Skeptical Inquirer 18:22–26, 56

Mackay C 1841 The magnetizers. In: Extraordinary popular delusions and the madness of crowds. Richard Bentley, London, reprinted in 1980 by Harmony Books, New York, pp. 304–345

Nadls S 1998 French scientist shrugs off winning his second Ig Nobel prize. Nature 395:535

Network 1999 Max Planck cited. Network 70:44

Pearson RD 1997 Consciousness as a sub-quantum phenomenon. Frontier Perspectives 6(2):70–78

Pert C 1997 Molecules of emotion. Scribner, New York, p 224

Pilla AA, Kaufman JJ, Ryaby JT 1987 Electrochemical kinetics at the cell membrane: a physicochemical link for electromagnetic bioeffects. In: Blank M, Findl E (eds) Mechanistic approaches to interactions of electric and electromagnetic fields with living systems. Plenum Press, New York, pp. 39–62

Stryer L 1987 The molecules of visual excitation. Scientific American, July, 42–50

Ueno S (ed)1996 Biological effects of magnetic and electromagnetic fields. Plenum Press, New York

Wiener N 1948 Cybernetics. Wiley, New York (2nd edn, 1961, MIT Press, Cambridge).

Westerhoff et al 1987 In: Blank M, Findl E (eds) Mechanistic approaches to interactions of electric and electromagnetic fields with living systems. Plenum Press, New York, pp. 203–215

Wilson W 1999 The new physics of CRI (the cranial rhythmic impulse). International Journal of Alternative and Complementary Medicine 17(8):6–9

Winter A 1998 Mesmerized. Powers of mind in Victorian Britain. University of Chicago Press, Chicago

Woodhouse MB 1996 Paradigm wars. Worldviews for a new age. Frog, Berkeley, CA, pp. 4–10

Zewail AH 1999 Studies of the transition states of chemical reactions using femtosecond spectroscopy. Nobel Prize in Chemistry, Karolinska Institutet.

Appendix I
Sources of gaussmeters and other EMF detectors

AlphaLab, Inc.
1280 South 300 West
Salt Lake City, UT 84101
USA
Tel: (USA or Canada): 1-800-769-3754
Tel: (elsewhere): 801-487-9492
E-mail: trifield@aros.net

DRUSCH GmbH.
Altenbekener Damm 51
D-30173 Hannover
Germany
Tel: +49-511-804615
web: http://www.drusch.com/
E-mail: webmaster@drusch.com

Holaday Industries, Inc.
14825 Martin Drive
Eden Prairie, MN 55344
USA
Tel: 612-934-4920

Magnetic Instrumentation Inc.
8431 Castlewood Drive
Indianapolis, IN 46250-1534
USA
Tel: 317-842-7500
Fax: 317-849-7600
E-mail: maginst@maginst.com

Magnetic Sciences
367 Arlington Street
Acton, MA 01720
USA
Tel: 1-978-266-9906
Fax: 1-978-266-9806
Email: mail@magneticsciences.com

Walker Scientific, Inc.
Rockdale Street
Worcester, MA 01606
USA
Tel: 508-852-3674
FAX: 508-856-9931
E-mail: info@walkerscientific.com
Web: www.walkermagnet.com

Appendix II
Books and articles on the health effects of electromagnetic pollution

Bennett WR 1995 Electromagnetic fields and power lines. Scientific American Science and Medicine 2(4):68–77

Blank M (ed) 1995 Electromagnetic Fields: biological interactions and mechanisms. Advances in Chemistry Series, 250. American Chemical Society, Washington DC

Bridges JE, Preache M 1981 Biological influences of power frequency electric fields: a tutorial review from a physical and experimental viewpoint. Proceedings of the IEEE 69:1092–1120

Brodeur P 1977 The zapping of America: microwaves, their deadly risk, and the cover up. Norton, New York

Brodeur P 1989 Currents of death: power lines, computer terminals, and the attempt to cover up their threat to your health. Simon & Schuster, New York

Brodeur P 1993 The great power-line cover-up: how the utilities and the government are trying to hide the cancer hazard posed by electromagnetic fields. Little, Brown, Boston

Carpenter DO, Ayrapetyan S (eds) 1994 Biological effects of electric and magnetic fields, Vol 1. Sources and mechanisms. Academic Press, San Diego

Carpenter DO, Ayrapetyan S (eds) 1994 Biological effects of electric and magnetic fields, Vol 2. Beneficial and harmful effects. Academic Press, San Diego

Committee on the Possible Effects of Electromagnetic Fields on Biological Systems 1997 Possible health effects of exposure to residential electric and magnetic fields. National Academy Press, Washington DC

De Merritt L 1990 Siting of power lines and communication towers: a bibliography on the potential health effects of electric and magnetic fields. Council of Planning Librarians, Chicago IL

Gandhi OP 1990 Biological effects and medical applications of electromagnetic fields. Prentice Hall, Englewood Cliffs, NJ

Grant L 1995 The electrical sensitivity handbook: how electromagnetic fields (Emfs) are making people sick. Weldon, Prescott, AZ

Horton WF, Goldberg S 1995 Power frequency magnetic fields and public health. CRC Press, Boca Raton

House of Representatives, One Hundred Second Congress, second session, March 10, 1992 National Electromagnetic Fields Research and Public Information Dissemination Act: hearing before the Subcommittee on Environment of the Committee on Science, Space, and Technology

House of Representatives, One Hundred Third Congress, first session 1993 Electric and magnetic fields: hearing before the Subcommittee on Energy and Power of the Committee on Energy and Commerce

International Radiation Protection Association. International Non-ionising Radiation Committee 1993 Protection of workers from power frequency electric and magnetic fields: a practical guide. Occupational Safety and Health Series, No. 69. International Labor Office, Geneva

Levitt BB 1995 Electromagnetic fields: a consumer's guide to the issues and how to protect ourselves. Harcourt Brace, San Diego

Nordén B, Ramel C 1992 Interaction mechanisms of low-level electromagnetic fields in living systems. Oxford University Press, New York

Pinsky MA 1995 The EMF book: what you should know about electromagnetic fields, electromagnetic radiation, and your health. Warner Books, New York

Polk C, Postow E (eds) 1996 Handbook of biological effects of electromagnetic fields, 2nd edn. CRC Press, Boca Raton.

Prata S 1993 Emf handbook: understanding and controlling electromagnetic fields in your life. Waite Group Press, Corte Madera, CA

Sugarman E 1992 Warning – the electricity around you may be hazardous to your health: how to protect yourself from electromagnetic fields. Simon & Schuster, New York

Swartwout G 1991 Electromagnetic Pollution Solutions. Aerai Publications, Hilo, HI

Tarkan L 1994 Electromagnetic fields: what you need to know to protect your health. Foreword by A.R. Liboff. Bantam Books, New York

Ueno S 1996 Biological effects of magnetic and electromagnetic fields. Plenum Press, New York

Wilson BW, Stevens RG, Anderson LE 1990 Extremely low frequency electromagnetic fields: the question of cancer. Battelle Press, Columbus

Index